TOP

5

QUESTIONS
TO ASK
YOUR
DOCTOR

TOP 5 QUESTIONS TO ASK YOUR DOCTOR

Important questions your doctor wants you to ask about your medical condition

JIM SUTTON, RPA-C

SAGAR NIGWEKAR, MD

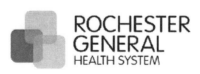
ROCHESTER GENERAL HEALTH SYSTEM

Outskirts Press, Inc.
Denver, Colorado

The information provided in this book is for informational purposes only and is not intended to be specific medical advice for the reader. Using this book does not create a professional doctor/patient relationship between the reader and the authors. This book is not intended to replace the services of a licensed professional and readers should consult their doctor in all matters related to their health.

About the Authors

Jim Sutton, RPA-C has been a practicing Family Practice Physician Assistant for 23 years. He graduated from the University of Washington Physician Assistant program in 1987 and also a residency in Pediatrics at Yale School of Medicine in 1993. He has spent his career serving vulnerable underserved patients in Los Angeles, the Middle East, and now in urban Rochester, NY for the Rochester General Health System. He is an Adjunct Clinical Professor for the Rochester Institute of Technology and he teaches Physician Assistant students in Family Medicine at Clinton Family Health Center in Rochester. His area of interest is health care policy and development of programs that target healthcare disparities.

Sagar Nigwekar, MD is a practicing Board Certified Internal Medicine physician at Rochester General Hospital. He graduated from the University of Mumbai, India in 1999 and subsequently completed his post-graduate training at the Rochester General Hospital Internal Medicine Residency Program. He was a Chief Medical Resident at Rochester General Hospital in 2005. Since then he has been teaching medical students and resident physicians at the University of Rochester School of Medicine and Dentistry. He has recently been selected to attend Brigham and Women's Hospital/Massachusetts General Hospital Joint Nephrology Fellowship Program (Harvard Medical School). He conducts translational and clinical research in the areas of hypertension and kidney diseases.

Dedication

I want to thank my beautiful wife Maria and my daughters Mila and Marisela for all the support and patience they gave me during my long nights working on this book.

– Jim Sutton

I would like to dedicate this book to my father Dr Uday Nigwekar, a lifetime patient advocate and a master communicator. I would also like to thank my wonderful and always supportive family members- Rosy, Nanda, Nirmal, Radhika and Sarabjit.

– Sagar Nigwekar

We would both like to thank all the physicians, physician assistants, medical students, and patients that unselfishly gave their time and effort reviewing this book and offering questions.

– Jim and Sagar

Table of Contents

How to Use this Book

Every minute of every day, in thousands of medical office visits, there is information people should know about their medical condition that is not being discussed. There are so many reasons for this phenomenon that they are too numerous to even list. The reality is that critical information is not being passed along to patients.

To avoid this situation and to help both patients and doctors have better conversations we have created this book of the top 5 questions you should ask your doctor about your medical condition. These questions have been submitted and reviewed by hundreds of primary care doctors, specialists, nurses, medical students, and patients. We believe if you ask these 5 simple questions at the time of your office visit you will have covered the "basics" of your medical condition.

We have intentionally left out the answers to these questions so your doctor can individualize the response as it applies to your particular situation. To help start the conversation we have also given you a brief overview of the medical condition at the beginning of each section. This overview is written in generalities, and some of it may not apply directly to your situation, so we encourage you to discuss the paragraph with your doctor to see if any of that information applies to you.

In this book we have used the generic word "doctor" to encompass any medical provider that is licensed to practice medicine such as a physician assistant, nurse practitioner, or nurse mid-wife.

You may want to begin this book by reading the *"Tips for Talking to Your Doctor"* section first. You then might want to read the *"Questions You Should Ask at Every Visit"* section to learn about general questions that apply to every visit. Next, reading *"Questions You Should Ask About Your Medications"* would be very helpful since most modern day medical visits result in a medication being prescribed. After that, we have included two sections that apply to special circumstances - *"Questions You Should Ask When in the Hospital,"* and *"Questions You Should Ask Before a Surgery or a Procedure."* You can use these sections if they apply to your particular circumstances or just skip them and go to whatever medical condition applies to you.

We encourage you to bring this book with you to each office visit to discuss your individual diagnosis with your doctor. In fact, better yet, ask your doctor to place some copies of the book in his/her examination rooms so all patients could benefit from these questions.

If you don't find a medical condition listed in this book, we encourage you to visit our website (www.top5questions.net) and post your condition. We would love to share with you questions about that condition and we encourage our patients to ask us about conditions that are not listed in this book.

We wish you the best of luck and the best of health.

Jim Sutton, RPA-C
Sagar Nigwekar, MD

Tips for Talking to Your Doctor

Entering a doctor's office can be like entering a different world. There are often "rules" and "protocols" that the doctor, nurses, and staff follow that you may not be familiar with. This book offers some very helpful questions for you to have an intelligent conversation with your doctor, but there are other things that can be helpful in making the office visit better.

When you think about the patient/doctor relationship, the word "relationship" is very important. The typical doctor has 2000 to 3000 patients, most of whom they see only once or twice a year. Seeing 20 to 30 of these patients each day, most doctors have only professional relationships with their patients and the majority of their patients are known by just a name and whatever information is in the medical record. This is worsened by the fact that you may only see your doctor for a few minutes a couple times a year. Therefore, you should be in "relationship building" mode from the minute you enter the office. The better the relationship you have with your primary doctor, the higher the likelihood you can have good and detailed conversations with him or her.

What do we mean by "relationship building?" Well, think of any relationship you have with people close to you and what you do to build those relationships. Think of your spouse, co-workers, casual friends, and family and the things you do to have good relationships with these people. Those same basic principles can go a long way to help build a relationship with your doctor. Here are a few tips.

Dress for success

Dressing professionally shows power and confidence. Doctors and their staff are people too, and even though you shouldn't judge a book by its cover, we all do! If you were going for an interview, going to the bank to ask for a loan, or going out on a date for the first time you would try to look your best to make a good first impression. Dress up to see your doctor, and you will see the difference in your treatment at every step of the visit.

Bring someone with you

Doctors are used to having more than one person in the room at a time. A doctor will act differently with more than one person in the room, because most people function differently in group settings than one-on-one. Also, when you are sick or dealing with an uncomfortable diagnosis, having another person in the room to remember what was said is always helpful. Whoever comes with you can sometimes catch things from the conversation that you may have missed. One word of caution: make sure you are comfortable discussing personal information in front of the person you bring!

Connect with your doctor

Building a relationship is about connecting with the other person. Doctors normally allow a minute or two at the beginning of the visit for this connection. Take this time to smile, shake hands, make good eye contact, and use this time to "socialize" before the visit begins. Good opening lines are "Looks like a busy day today" or "I haven't seen you in a long time" or "I like the changes you made to the waiting room."

Set the agenda

Doctors have a limited amount of time for office visits. In order to use their time wisely they usually set the agenda and control the visit as much as possible. Because of this control you may realize that the visit is over before you got around to asking your questions. To prevent this, be involved in setting the agenda for the visit. Most doctors will start the visit with an opening question such as "How can I help you today?" or "What can I do for you today?" This is your opportunity to set the agenda. If you say, "I have had this headache for three days," then the doctor will shift their brain into headache mode and that becomes the agenda for the day. Here are some ways to set the agenda:

Doctor: How can I help you today?

Patient: I am not sick today. I just want to spend a few minutes talking about my diabetes, and I have some questions to ask you about my illness.

Doctor: How can I help you today?

Patient: I have had a headache for three days. After you make your diagnosis, I would like to ask you a couple questions about my condition.

Most doctors consider the diagnosis as the end of the visit and then shift their attention to prescribing a treatment. If you don't warn your doctor that you are going to finish the visit with a few questions, then he/she may not time the visit correctly and the visit may start to run overtime as you ask your questions.

Use your time wisely

Timing is everything. Be prepared to talk about your questions and issues in the least amount of time. Have your questions ready before the doctor enters the room. If you are there for a specific symptom, then as soon as a diagnosis (or possible diagnosis) is mentioned, open your book to the appropriate page and be prepared to ask your questions.

Allow for some silence

A well timed pause goes a long way. How many times have you tried to get something done while someone else is chatting away and breaking your concentration? Don't ask your questions during the examination, or when the prescription is being written, or if the doctor is still asking questions to determine the diagnosis. Let the conversation flow naturally and allow the doctor time to "practice his/her craft" such as look in the record, perform an examination, and ask questions. Save your questions for after this is done.

Questions You Should Ask at Every Visit

There are certain questions that are important to ask anytime you see your doctor. It is important to know and understand what your health problems are, as well as to understand your treatment. If your doctor has recently diagnosed a new medical condition, or is starting or changing a treatment, you will find these questions very helpful. In addition to the disease-specific questions in this book, you should also ask these questions about your treatment whenever you can.

Top 5 questions-

How will I know that my treatment is working?

How will the medication or treatment you are prescribing treat my condition?

Is there more than one condition that could be causing my problem?

What exactly is my condition, and what caused it?

What symptoms should I look for that means I should contact you or seek immediate help?

Additional questions you may consider asking-

Are there treatment choices that don't involve medications?

How long will it take for me to feel better?

If my symptoms get worse, what can I do on my own before I see you?

Is my medical condition permanent or temporary?

Questions You Should Ask About Your Medications

Any time you are prescribed a medicine you should ask these questions:

Top 5 questions-

Can I take a generic medicine or is this available over the counter?

Can you review my instructions with me?
- At what time should I take this medication?
- Should I take it with or without food?
- Can I take it with other medications?

What are the possible risks and side effects of this medication?

What is the reason for taking this medication, and how does it work?

Will this medication interact with any other medication I am taking?

Additional questions you may consider asking-

Can my medication be stopped suddenly or does it need to be stopped slowly?

Do I need to follow any restrictions (alcohol, driving, and work)?

Do you think a pill box will help me?

How long will I need to take my medicine?

If I do not tolerate this medication then what are my alternatives?

What should I do if I miss a dose?

Where do I store this medication at home?

Questions You Should Ask When in the Hospital

A hospital stay can be overwhelming and knowing what to expect and what to ask will make your stay in the hospital less stressful.

Who is in charge?

Your own doctor may have advised you to go to the hospital but that doesn't always mean your doctor will take care of you while you are there. You might have one doctor in charge of your overall care (a *hospitalist* that specializes in taking care of people in the hospital) and likely a couple of specialists also involved. This team will contact your doctor and discuss the plan for care, but in some cases your doctor may not see you while you are in the hospital. It is important to ask your primary care doctor who will be taking care of you in case you are hospitalized, and make sure you know their name.

Top 5 questions-

Are you in touch with my primary care doctor?

Do you know what medicines I take at home?

Have any of my home medications been stopped, and why?

How long will I need to stay in the hospital?

Who should I follow up with after my hospitalization?

Additional questions you may consider asking-

What time of the day will you see me, and how do I reach you in-between? How do my family members reach you?

Which tests are being ordered and why? When will I get the results of these tests?

Questions You Should Ask Before Surgery or a Procedure

Every day thousands of patients have surgery or other types of medical procedures. It is important to know some basic information about the surgery or procedure so you can make a better choice as to whether or not it is the right thing for you, and you can be better prepared when the time comes for the surgery. Below are some questions you may want to ask your doctor prior to any procedure or surgery.

Top 5 questions-

How long will I be in the hospital after this procedure/surgery?

Is this an urgent procedure/surgery, or can it be done later (elective)?

What are the possible risks of this procedure/surgery?

What is the exact reason for this procedure/surgery?

What things can I expect during recovery?

Additional questions you may consider asking-

How long will this procedure/surgery last?

What do I need to do to prepare for this procedure/surgery?

What type of anesthesia will I receive?

What other treatments will be necessary after the procedure/surgery?

Who will be doing this procedure/surgery, and how many of these procedures has the doctor done?

Will I be awake during this procedure/surgery?

Abdominal Aortic Aneurysm (AAA or Triple A)

An abdominal aortic aneurysm is the stretching of the large blood vessel (aorta) that runs down the middle of the abdomen (belly). A normal size for an abdominal aorta is about ½ inch in diameter. In time, and if a person is a smoker or has a lot of plaques in their arteries (atherosclerosis) the wall of the aorta can weaken and stretch out like a balloon. Often the doctor can feel it when they are examining the abdomen. If the AAA is small (less than 2 inches in diameter), not painful, and not growing fast, it sometimes does not need be repaired. Decisions about repairing an AAA surgically are made on an individual basis.

Top 5 questions-

Do I need a special test such as an abdominal ultrasound or CAT scan?

In my specific case, do I need to have my AAA repaired?

Should I avoid any contact sports or strenuous activities like lifting?

Since I have an AAA, does that mean I can have aneurysms in other parts of my body?

What caused my AAA?

Additional questions you may consider asking-

Should other people in my family be tested for this?

What is the risk of surgery verses not doing anything at all?

Addison's Disease

Addison's disease is also called primary adrenal insufficiency. With this condition your adrenal glands (small glands sitting on top of your kidneys) don't make enough hormones (chemicals). The adrenal glands make hormones that help you cope with stress. Addison's disease can cause a decreased appetite and weight loss, mood changes, dizziness, nausea, and fatigue. It also can cause brown patches or darkening of areas of the skin around the nipples, back of neck, and areas where the skin folds on itself. It is usually treated with steroids or hormone replacement therapy.

Top 5 questions-

Is there anything I can do or take for the symptoms?

What are some of the symptoms I can expect from Addison's disease?

What are the long-term risks of having Addison's disease?

What is my hormone level and how does that compare to normal?

What is the adrenal stimulation test and why is it necessary to do this test?

Additional questions you may consider asking-

Can Addison's disease cause changes in my sexual desire?

Can I get the brown patches in my mouth?

Do I need to see a specialist (endocrinologist)?

Is there anyway I can do to make the brown patches on my skin go away?

Will this ever go away or will it last my whole life?

AIDS (HIV)

HIV stands for human immunodeficiency virus. If you are infected with this virus you will have it for the rest of your life. AIDS stands for acquired immune deficiency syndrome and it is the medical condition that happens as a result of having the HIV virus. With newer medications available today, many people have the HIV virus but don't go on to get AIDS. With AIDS you have difficulty fighting off certain germs and can develop infections (and certain cancers) that can be very serious. It is important that people that are HIV positive (have the HIV virus) treat their condition with anti-viral medications to prevent getting these serious infections.

Top 5 questions-

How is HIV not spread?

How is HIV spread from person to person?

What are the infections I can get because I have AIDS?

What is my HIV viral load and CD4 count and what does that tell me about my illness?

What is my T-cell count?

Additional questions you may consider asking-

Am I contagious (can pass this to another person)?

Am I required to notify anybody that I am HIV positive (work, school, athletic facility)?

Are there any support groups I could attend and do you suggest any counseling for me?

Do I need to see a specialist for my care?

How often should I see a doctor and get a blood test?

If I am pregnant, can I deliver my baby? How can I protect my baby from HIV?

If I am seeing a specialist for my care, what do I do if I have a routine medical problem? Who do I see?

Should I avoid breast feeding if I have HIV?

What are the advantages or disadvantages of starting anti-viral medications sooner than later?

What are the chances that my sexual partner can become infected with HIV if we use condoms?

What things can I do to keep my immune system as healthy as possible?

Will I need to take my medications for the rest of my life?

Alcohol Dependence and Withdrawal (Alcoholism)

Alcohol dependence (also known as alcoholism) is a chronic (over a long time) and severe drinking problem. It happens when you drink alcohol too much or too often over a long period of time. With alcoholism you crave alcohol, cannot stop yourself from drinking, and the affects of alcohol disrupt your normal daily routines (work, school, family). Withdrawing from alcohol can cause very dangerous effects to your body and at times can be life-threatening.

Top 5 questions-

Are there any medications that can prevent me from drinking?

I have a family history of alcoholism. Does that put me at increased risk?

What are the signs I am dependent upon alcohol?

What do my liver function tests show?

Would Alcoholics Anonymous (or a similar program) be appropriate for me?

Additional questions you may consider asking-

Do I need to be admitted into a treatment facility to withdrawal from the effects of alcohol?

Do I need to see a specialist (substance abuse doctor or counselor)?

What are withdrawal signs and symptoms?

Alopecia

Alopecia is hair loss, but not the natural hair loss that comes with aging. There are generally two types of alopecia. Alopecia areata is patches of hair loss and is the most common form of hair loss not related to normal balding. Alopecia totalis is complete hair loss and is very rare (only occurring in about 1% of cases). Alopecia usually only affects the scalp and beard area but sometimes can affect eyebrows and other areas of the body. Alopecia can sometimes run in the family. In most cases it is a self limiting condition. That is, it will eventually go away on its own after a period of time.

Top 5 questions-

Are there any other medical conditions that could be causing my alopecia?

How long, on average, will it take for my hair to grow back?

Is my alopecia contagious (can be passed to another person)?

The area of hair loss tingles. Is that normal?

Will I get more patches of hair loss besides the ones I have now?

Additional questions you may consider asking-

Are there other treatment choices besides medications?

Can this happen again?

Is it necessary that I see a skin specialist (dermatologist)?

What is the natural course of this disorder (how it progresses)?

Will minoxidil (Rogaine - a lotion you apply to your scalp to grow hair) work on my hair loss patches?

Amenorrhea

Amenorrhea is when a woman fails to have menstrual periods. The condition is known as "primary amenorrhea" when a woman has never menstruated; and "secondary amenorrhea" if her periods stop after having been regular for months or years. The most common cause of amenorrhea is pregnancy, and this should always be excluded before other possible causes are considered. Increased exercise and stress can also cause amenorrhea. Certain medications as well as hormone deficiencies or conditions with the pituitary gland can also cause amenorrhea.

Top 5 questions-

Are there any medications that can make my periods regular again?

Do any tests need to be done to determine the cause of my amenorrhea?

What, in your opinion, is the cause of my amenorrhea?

What is likely to happen if I don't treat my amenorrhea?

What treatments do you recommend?

Additional questions you may consider asking-

Has pregnancy been ruled-out as a possible cause of my amenorrhea?

How long should I wait without having a period before I contact you?

Is it dangerous to not have menstrual periods?

Anal Fissure (Anal Tear)

An anal fissure is a tear on the inside of the anus. The anus is the opening where stool from your bowel movements leave the body. Tears can come from constipation, pushing too hard during bowel movements, infections, or trauma. Anal fissures can be very painful. First time small tears can heal by themselves but if the tear is large or happens over again it may need correction by surgery.

Top 5 questions-

Are there any changes I can make in my diet to help this condition?

Do I need a biopsy? What does a biopsy involve?

Do I need surgery?

How much water should I drink per day to prevent constipation?

What are the risks of treating this surgically?

Additional questions you may consider asking-

Can this happen again?

Can this heal on its own without treatment?

Sometimes I see blood in my stool, is that normal?

What are the benefits of treating this with medications verses surgery?

What is a Sitz bath and how do I perform it at home? Will it help my symptoms?

Anemia

Anemia is when your blood lacks enough healthy red blood cells. Red blood cells are the main transporters of oxygen in your body. The symptom of anemia is fatigue. Women, and people with chronic diseases, are at increased risk for anemia. Also, there are certain forms of anemia that run in the family and infants may be affected with those forms of anemia from birth. Women are particularly susceptible to a form of anemia called iron-deficiency anemia because of blood loss from menstruation. Older people may have a greater risk of getting anemia because of a poor diet and other medical conditions. Iron-deficiency anemia is the most common type and can usually be treated with dietary changes and iron supplements. In all, there are more than 400 different types of anemia.

Top 5 questions-

Are there any dietary changes I can make to treat my anemia?

Could my anemia be caused by some other medical condition?

What blood tests do I need to find out the type of anemia I have?

What is my hemoglobin count and what is the meaning of that number?

What is my red blood cell count and what is the meaning of that number?

Additional questions you may consider asking-

Can taking iron supplements cause constipation?

What are the symptoms that mean I have a more series medical condition?

What foods are naturally high in iron?

Will taking a daily vitamin help my anemia?

Angina

Angina is pain in the chest you feel from lack of oxygen in your coronary arteries (the blood vessels that supply blood to the wall of the heart). It is not a "heart attack", but people that suffer from angina are at risk to have a heart attack. The lack of oxygen to the blood vessels can happen from blockage of blood vessels or from a spasm. Blockage usually happens from having high cholesterol.

Top 5 questions-

What do I look for that means I need to go to the hospital immediately?

What are some daily activities that can cause angina?

What lifestyle changes can I make to lower my risk of getting angina?

What things put me at risk for having angina?

What type of angina do I have? (stable, unstable, Prinzmental's or variant, microvascular, atypical)

Additional questions you may consider asking-

Do I need a cardiac catherization (a camera passed into the heart) or an echocardiogram (an ultrasound of the heart)?

How is my angina diagnosed?

I get a headache when I take my nitroglycerin; is that normal?

Is my angina being caused by a blockage or a spasm?

What is the difference between stable and unstable angina?

Will controlling my blood pressure help my symptoms?

Ankylosing Spondylitis

Ankylosing spondylitis is a long-term condition that causes back pain, neck pain or hip pain and stiffness. This condition is caused by the joining together (ankylosing) and inflammation (spondylitis) of bones in the spine. The exact cause of ankylosing spondylitis is not known, but certain genetic conditions are thought to be associated with this condition.

Top 5 questions-

Am I likely to need surgery for ankylosing spondylitis?

Do I need a genetic test for this condition?

Do I need any tests such as x-rays at this time?

What are the possible risks of having ankylosing spondylitis?

What other conditions have the same symptoms as ankylosing spondylitis?

Additional questions you may consider asking-

Can ankylosing spondylitis involve body parts other than the spine?

Can you recommend any home exercises for this condition?

Do my family members need to be tested for this condition?

Do you think physical therapy will help this condition?

Is my ankylosing spondylitis likely to get worse over time?

Should I take calcium and vitamin D supplements?

What can I do to prevent ankylosing spondylitis from getting worse?

Anxiety

Anxiety is a common medical condition. Doctors will often call this condition General Anxiety Disorder or GAD. It is characterized by excessive worry about everyday things and at times can be disabling as it begins to interfere with daily activities such as work, school or relationships. There can be a variety of symptoms for anxiety such as trembling, insomnia (difficulty falling asleep), sweating, irritability, difficulty concentrating, and sometimes chest tightness or the inability to catch your breath. This condition is often treated with anti-anxiety medications that can either be taken at the time of symptoms or taken daily to prevent symptoms.

Top 5 questions-

Could my anxiety be caused by another medical condition?

Should I see a specialist (psychiatrist or counselor)?

What is the best thing to do when I have an anxiety attack?

When can I expect this to go away?

When my pulse races, how do I know it is not a heart condition?

Additional questions you may consider asking-

Are there substances I should avoid, or lifestyle changes I should make?

Can relaxation therapy or bio-therapy help?

How long should I take medications, and can I become addicted to them?

How often can I take my anti-anxiety medications?

What are some of the side effects of anti-anxiety medications?

Appendicitis

Appendicitis is inflammation or infection of the appendix. The appendix is a small pouch attached to the large intestine. Appendicitis is rare before age two and most commonly happens between ages 10 and 30, although anyone can suffer from this. Once the inflamed appendix becomes infected it is an urgent medical condition. Classic symptoms of an appendicitis is a dull pain that starts at the navel and then becomes sharp and moves to the lower right side of the abdomen, loss of appetite and nausea or vomiting, abdominal (belly) swelling, and fever.

Top 5 questions-

Can I expect any long-term consequences from appendicitis?

Can I take any medications for the pain or fever?

How is appendicitis diagnosed?

Is this an emergency?

Should I eat or drink anything while I am waiting for the final diagnosis or surgery?

Additional questions you may consider asking-

Can this happen again?

How long will I be in the hospital?

How long will it take for me to recover from the surgery?

Arrhythmias (Abnormal Heart Beats)

An arrhythmia is a medical term used to describe conditions associated with abnormal heart rhythms. A variety of conditions such as heart disease, certain chemical imbalances in your body (such as low potassium or magnesium), and conditions such as infections can cause arrhythmias. There are specific names for some arrhythmias you may hear your doctor mention such as; premature ventricular contractions, premature atrial contractions, atrial flutter, atrial fibrillation, tachycardia and bradycardia. Arrhythmias can cause palpitations (pounding in the chest), chest pain, and shortness of breath or dizziness.

Top 5 questions-

Do I need to be on a blood thinner such as aspirin or warfarin?

What is the cause of my arrhythmia?

What symptoms can I experience because of this arrhythmia?

What tests do I need to have to determine the cause of my arrhythmia?

What type of arrhythmia do I have?

Additional questions you may consider asking-

Is my arrhythmia a short-term condition or is it likely to last longer?

What are the possible risks from having arrhythmias?

What lifestyle changes do you recommend to improve my arrhythmia?

Which activities should I avoid because of my arrhythmia?

Will I benefit from a pacemaker or a defibrillator?

Arthralgia (Joint Pain)

This is a common medical condition that can involve one or more joints (such as the knees, hips, elbows, shoulders, or small joints like the hands and feet) and can be caused by a variety of conditions such as osteoarthritis (wear and tear of joints), trauma to the joints (sprain), and immune conditions such as rheumatoid arthritis or lupus. Pain in the joints can also be caused by damage to bones, cartilage or ligaments and sometimes it can be a referred pain, that is, pain starting in one joint that radiates to another joint. In most cases, joint pain will go away in a short time, but if it is caused by a chronic medical condition such as osteoarthritis it may last longer.

Top 5 questions-

Can you recommend any home exercises or physical therapy for my joint pain?

Do I need any tests such as an x-ray or blood tests to find out more about my joint pain?

What is the cause of my joint pain?

Which activities should I avoid because of my joint pain?

Which medicines do you recommend for this pain?
- Are any of these medications available over the counter?

Additional questions you may consider asking-

Can I apply heat or ice to my painful joints?

Do I need a surgery or a joint steroid injection treatment?

Do I need to see a specialist (orthopedician or rheumatologist)?

Do you recommend using any special orthoses (shoe inserts or splints) or supports (cane)?

How long do you think my joint pain will last?

If my joint pain or swelling gets worse when starting exercise, what should I do?

Is my joint pain likely to get worse with time?

Once my joint pain goes away, am I likely to get this pain again?

What can I do to prevent this condition from deteriorating (getting worse)?

What other symptoms am I likely to develop because of my arthralgias?

Arthritis

Arthritis (inflammation of the joints) causes painful, swollen, and stiff joints. There are many different causes of arthritis and they can involve one or many joints at the same time. Osteoarthritis (degenerative joint disease or wear and tear arthritis) is the most common type of arthritis. Rheumatoid arthritis, lupus arthritis, psoriatic arthritis and gout are some of the other causes of arthritis.

Top 5 questions-

Do I need any tests such as x-rays or blood tests to confirm the diagnosis?

Is my arthritis likely to affect other parts of my body (such as liver, skin)?

What is the cause of my arthritis?

Which medications do you recommend for arthritis?
- Can I take over the counter pain medications for arthritis pain?

What type of arthritis do I have?

Additional questions you may consider asking-

Are my family members at risk for getting my type of arthritis?

Can I apply heat or cold to my painful joints?

Can you suggest any home exercises for arthritis?

Do I need a referral to see a specialist (orthopedician or rheumatologist)?

Do you recommend using any special orthoses (such as shoe inserts or splints) and supports (such as a cane)?

Do you think my arthritis is related to any previous joint injury?

If my joint pain or swelling gets worse with exercise what should I do?

Is my arthritis likely to get worse with time?

Should I avoid certain activities or joint movements?

Should I have any restrictions at work or school because of my arthritis?

What are some of the risks of having arthritis?

What can I do to prevent arthritis?

What can I do to prevent my arthritis from deteriorating (getting worse)?

What other symptoms am I likely to develop because of this condition?

Will I benefit from a joint replacement surgery?

Will I benefit from seeing a physical therapist or an occupational therapist? If yes, should I see them prior to starting any home exercises?

Asthma

Asthma is a common medical condition caused by inflammation of the airways. People with asthma have difficulty breathing, cough, wheezing or chest tightness. There are a variety of triggers (exercise, allergens, infection) that can make asthma symptoms worse. Asthma can run in the family. Asthma is treated with medications that relax the airway muscles (bronchodilators) and medications that reduce inflammation (corticosteroids, leukotriene inhibitors).

Top 5 questions-

Can you show me how to use my inhaler correctly?

How often can I use a rescue inhaler?

How often should I get pulmonary function tests to monitor my asthma?

How severe is my asthma?

What are the possible triggers of my asthma and how can I avoid them?

Additional questions you may consider asking-

Can my wheezing be from another medical condition?

Do I need to make any changes to my home or work place?

I have a heart condition. What asthma medications should I avoid?

If I am pregnant, are all asthma medications safe to use?

Should I be using a daily medication in addition to my rescue inhaler?

Should I have an annual flu shot or a pneumonia shot every 5 years?

Atherosclerosis

Atherosclerosis is a medical condition caused by an increase of fats in the wall of blood vessels. This build up of fats can eventually lead to complications such as heart attacks, angina, stroke, kidney disease and peripheral vascular disease. There are a number of risk factors for atherosclerosis like high blood pressure (hypertension), diabetes, high cholesterol (hyperlipidemia), tobacco use and advancing age. The good news is that many of these risk factors are treatable and some are preventable all together.

Top 5 questions-

Are there medications that can lower my risk of atherosclerosis?

Do I need any additional tests at this time?

How extensive is my atherosclerosis, and which body parts are involved?

What are the risk factors causing my atherosclerosis?

What do you recommend for managing these risk factors?

Additional questions you may consider asking-

Do my family members also need to be tested for atherosclerosis?

How do I get monitored for this condition?

How much is the blockage in my blood vessels?

Is atherosclerosis reversible?

What are some of the risks of atherosclerosis, and how can I lower them?

What is my cholesterol number? What is considered normal?

Attention Deficit Disorder (ADD)

ADD is a common medical condition that is seen in school aged children and sometimes adults. When combined with hyperactivity, it is known as ADHD (Attention Deficit-Hyperactivity Disorder). The main symptoms of ADD are difficulty paying attention, concentrating, controlling actions, and poor school performance. It normally becomes more apparent when a child enters school because of the additional concentration that school requires. As a child grows older and develops better coping skills for concentration the medications become less necessary. Sometimes medications are needed in adulthood, especially if concentration is interfering with work and personal relationships.

Top 5 questions-

Are medications absolutely necessary?

Do I need to see a specialist (psychiatrist or psychologist)?

Does my child need to take ADD medications on the weekend or during school breaks?

Is there treatment for ADD that does not involve medication?

What are the risks of taking ADD medications?

Additional questions you may consider asking-

Are there any special tests that need to be performed?

Are there any support groups I can attend?

Can I expect my child to grow out of ADD?

Could other medical conditions be causing these symptoms?

How do I distinguish between ADD and just "bad" behavior?

How often should I see the doctor for this condition?

What is the best time of the day to take ADD medications?

Why is a blood pressure medication (clonidine) being prescribed if this is a behavioral disorder?

Why is it necessary to perform an EKG (electrocardiogram)?

Will my child have ADD the rest of their life?

Back Pain

This is one of the most common reasons for a doctor's visit. There are a lot of causes of back pain and the pain might involve different parts of the back. In some cases the pain might radiate to other parts of the body such as the legs. Back pain is usually due to conditions involving muscles, ligaments, or bones of the back, and in some cases it might be from conditions that involve organs such as the kidneys or pancreas. Most back pain is short-term and gets better in a few days to weeks. Back pain that does not get better in a few weeks is called chronic and can be very difficult to adequately control.

Top 5 questions-

Do I need to restrict any activities because of my pain?

How long do you think my back pain will last?

What is the cause of my back pain?

Which medications do you recommend to treat my pain?
- Are any of these medications available over the counter?

Which tests do you recommend to further evaluate my back pain?

Additional questions you may consider asking-

Am I likely to get back pain again?

Can I apply heat or ice to the back for pain relief?

Can you recommend some home exercises or physical therapy for my back pain?

Do I need a surgery or a steroid injection treatment?

Do I need to see a specialist for my back (neurologist, pain specialist or chiropractor)?

Do you recommend any specific sitting or sleeping positions to help my back pain?

Do you recommend using a back brace?

I have a history of cancer. Can my back pain be caused by cancer?

If my back pain gets worse when I start exercise, what should I do?

Is my back pain likely to get worse with time?

What can I do to prevent my back pain from deteriorating (getting worse)?

What type of pillow do you recommend to help my back pain?

Would I benefit from a muscle relaxant medication?

Bacterial Vaginosis

Bacterial vaginosis (often called BV) is an infection of the vagina and is one of the most common vaginal infections that affect women. It is not entirely known what causes bacterial vaginosis, but it is thought that the vagina has many good bacteria that prevent infection and when the normal balance of the vagina changes the amount of good bacteria can be too low and "bad" bacteria can take over causing BV. It is not a sexually transmitted disease. You are more likely to get BV if you are sexually active, douche frequently, or have an intrauterine device (IUD). Symptoms include vaginal discharge, burning and a "fishy" smell that sometimes is more prominent after intercourse. BV is treated with antibiotics in either a cream or pill form.

Top 5 questions-

Can I have sex during the time I am using the antibiotic cream?

Do you have any advice about the correct type of underwear or pantyhose that can help prevent BV? Should I use a special soap to avoid BV?

How often can I safely douche? In general, is douching necessary?

Should I abstain from intercourse during my treatment for BV?

Will the pills I am taking for BV cause a reaction if I drink alcohol?

Additional questions you may consider asking-

Can I tell this is BV by my symptoms?

Could my tampons be causing BV?

Does my partner need to be tested or treated?

Have you confirmed with your tests that this is not a STD?

Barrett's Esophagus

The esophagus is the food pipe that connects your mouth to the stomach. Sometimes because of repetitive damage to the esophagus from acid in the stomach (acid reflux), the esophagus lining gets replaced by a different cell type. This new lining increases the risk of getting cancer of the esophagus. Barrett's esophagus is usually diagnosed by a procedure called an endoscopy. Since this diagnosis has many implications, the diagnosis needs to be confirmed by at least two different doctors.

Top 5 questions-

How severe is the abnormality of the esophagus on the biopsy?

If I improve the acid reflux then is Barrett's esophagus reversible?

What are the risks of having Barrett's esophagus?

What do you recommend to manage this medical condition?

What is the cause of my Barrett's esophagus?

Additional questions you may consider asking-

Do I need to have an endoscopy every few months?

Do I need to have surgery to correct this condition?

Were my biopsy samples examined by a gastroenterological pathologist? Did two or more pathologists agree on the diagnosis?

What is the likelihood of developing cancer of the esophagus?

What measures do you recommend to prevent esophageal cancer?

Which foods make acid reflux worse?

Bell's Palsy

Bell's palsy is a temporary form of facial paralysis (inability to move the muscles) that happens when there is damage to the nerves that control the muscles of the face. Bell's palsy always happens on one side of the face and makes it difficult for one eye to blink and can make one side of the mouth droop. It is not associated with other symptoms like leg or arm paralysis. The exact cause of Bell's palsy is not known although sometimes it is caused by a virus that makes the nerves become temporarily inflamed. In most cases no treatment is necessary and the palsy will go away on its own in a few weeks.

Top 5 questions-

Are there any activities I should avoid?

How long will it take for the palsy to go away?

Is this a permanent condition?

Should I wear any eye protection until I am better?

What can I do if my eye gets extra dry?

Additional questions you may consider asking-

Are there any special exercises I can do to make the palsy go away faster?

Can this happen again?

Do I need any special tests?

Do I need to be started on medication to treat the virus?

How can I distinguish between Bell's palsy and a stroke?

Benign Prostatic Hypertrophy (BPH)

BPH is when the prostate gland grows in size. It is a nonmalignant (noncancerous) enlargement of the prostate gland, and a very common occurrence in older men (over 50), but sometimes can happen earlier in life. The larger size of the prostate compresses the urethra which can slow down the flow of urine. Common symptoms include a slow flow of urine, frequent urination, the need to urinate urgently and difficulty starting the urinary stream. More serious problems include urinary tract infections and complete blockage of the urethra, which can be a medical emergency and lead to injury of the kidneys. Treatment of BPH is usually reserved for men with significant symptoms. A simple blood test called a PSA can also be used for screening and most doctors recommend it be done annually in men over 50 and sooner if the man is at high risk of developing cancer of the prostate.

Top 5 questions-

Are there treatments for this condition that does not involve medicines?

Do I need to have a blood test (PSA)?

How often should I have my prostate checked?

When will I need to start medications for my BPH?

Will treatment affect my sexual function?

Additional questions you may consider asking-

Do I need a cystocopy?

What are the advantages and disadvantages of surgical treatment?

What is the normal amount of times a male in his 50's should urinate at night?

Bleeding Disorders

A variety of medical conditions and medications can increase your risk for bleeding. Bleeding disorders may present with bruises on the skin, "blood blisters" in the mouth, heavy menstrual periods, blood in the stool, blood in the urine, swollen joints, or excessive bleeding after a surgery or procedure. Common conditions that can cause this include hemophilia, Von Willebrand disease, low platelet count (thrombocytopenia) and inflammation of blood vessels (vasculitis). Medications such as prednisone, aspirin, naprosyn, ibuprofen, antibiotics and warfarin can also lead to increased bleeding.

Top 5 questions-

If I need a surgical procedure then what precautions should I take?

What tests do I need to have at this time? How often do I need these tests?

Which activities should I avoid?

Which medications should I avoid to reduce my bleeding risk?

Why do I bleed more than normal?

Additional questions you may consider asking-

Is this condition likely to last all my life?

Should other people in my family be tested for bleeding disorders?

What are some of the risks of having a bleeding disorder?

What is the chance that my family members have a similar condition?

Which foods should I avoid to reduce my bleeding risk?

Blurred Vision

There are many reasons for blurred vision. Most often blurred vision is related to eye problems such as presbyopia (near vision) or myopia (far vision) or in some cases more serious eye problems such as cataracts or glaucoma. Sometimes non-eye medical conditions can cause blurred vision such as diabetes, brain disturbances (stroke or TIA), or migraine headaches. There are also some medications that can cause blurred vision. Even contact lenses can sometimes scratch the cornea (the covering of the eye) and cause an abrasion which can lead to blurred vision. Because there are so many causes for blurred vision your doctor may need to perform multiple tests to find the root cause. If your doctor believes the blurred vision is eye related then a referral to an eye specialist (ophthalmologist) is all that is needed.

Top 5 questions-

Do I need to see an eye doctor (ophthalmologist) or can I see someone who prescribes glasses (optometrist)?

If the blurred vision is associated with pain, what does that mean?

Is my blurred vision dangerous?

What other symptoms should I look for that can help determine the source of my blurred vision?

Will my blurred vision go away with treatment?

Additional questions you may consider asking-

Do I need a CAT scan or an MRI?

My vision is blurred even when I wear my glasses, is that normal?

Bronchitis

Bronchitis is inflammation of the large airways (bronchi) that branch from the trachea and is usually caused by an infection, but sometimes is caused by irritation from inhaling gases, smoke, dust particles, or some types of pollution. In most cases the infection is from a virus and does not require antibiotic treatment. The symptom of bronchitis is a cough that can last up to three months. If the cough lasts beyond that time period then the bronchitis is classified as "chronic" and may require different treatment. In most cases the diagnosis can be made based on a simple examination, but sometimes an x-ray is needed to exclude pneumonia.

Top 5 questions-

Are there any treatments for this that do not involve medicines?

What are the symptoms I should look for that means this is more serious?

What is the best over the counter cough medicine for my bronchitis?

What is the cause of my bronchitis?

You prescribed an inhaler; does that mean that I have asthma?

Additional questions you may consider asking-

Do I need a chest x-ray?

I seem to cough more when I lay down at night. Why?

If my symptoms don't go away, how long should I wait to see you again?

Is my bronchitis contagious (can be passed to someone else)?

Will stopping smoking make my bronchitis go away?

Bursitis

Bursitis is inflammation of a bursa. A bursa is a tiny fluid-filled sac that acts as a cushion between tissues of the body, and there are 160 bursa sacs in the body. The major sacs are located in the shoulders, elbows, hips, and knees. A bursa can become inflamed from injury, infection, or a rheumatic condition (such as arthritis). You can do something as simple as lifting a bag of groceries to inflame a bursa, or get an infection of a bursa on the knee by scraping it on the ground. Bursitis is usually diagnosed by an examination that shows pain or tenderness with motion of the joint. Sometimes an x-ray will be done to look for other reasons for the pain. The treatment can range from taking an antibiotic; an oral anti-inflammatory and pain medication; or a cortisone medication.

Top 5 questions-

Are there specific side effects from the oral anti-inflammatory medications I should be aware of?

What are the advantages of an injection verses an oral medication?

What are the risks of a cortisone injection?

What over the counter medications are available to treat this bursitis?

Will heat or ice help when my joint is painful and swollen?

Additional questions you may consider asking-

I always get bursitis in the same joint. Is there any way of preventing this?

If I do nothing, will my bursitis get worse?

Should I limit any activities when the bursa is inflamed?

Will this come back?

C. Diff. (Clostridium Difficile) Infection

C. Diff. (short for Clostridium Difficile) is a bacteria that can be found on many surfaces in healthcare settings (bedpans, toilet seats, linens, telephones, stethoscopes). It is the most common infection acquired by people while they are in the hospital. C. Diff. can also be acquired outside of hospitals in the community. When a patient takes an antibiotic, it disrupts the normal protective layer of the colon and can allow C. Diff. to take over and grow, causing colitis (an inflammation of the colon). People with mild C. Diff. colitis have a low-grade fever and mild diarrhea. People with severe C. Diff. colitis have a high fever, severe diarrhea with blood, and severe abdominal cramps. Dehydration is common with severe C. Diff. colitis.

Top 5 questions-

Am I contagious (can pass this to other people)?

Am I likely to have this again?

Are anti-diarrhea medications safe to take with C. Diff. colitis?

How much water should I be drinking each day?

What are the warning signs my condition is getting worse?

Additional questions you may consider asking-

Can I take over the counter pain medicines for my pain and fever?

How long will it take for my diarrhea to go away?

Is yogurt good to take during the times I have diarrhea? If so, then how often should I eat it?

Why do I need to take more antibiotics to make this go away?

Cancer

Cancer begins in the cells of the body. Normally, your body forms new cells as you need them, and replaces old cells as they die. Sometimes this process goes wrong. New cells grow even when you don't need them, and old cells don't die when they should. This causes a build up of extra cells that can grow into a mass called a tumor. Tumors can be benign or malignant. Benign tumors aren't cancer and malignant tumors are cancer. Cells from malignant tumors can spread to other parts of the body. Most cancers are named by where they start. For example, lung cancer starts in the lung, and breast cancer starts in the breast. The spread of cancer from one part of the body to another is called metastasis. Metastasis means the cancer is more advanced. Treatment depends on the type of cancer and how far it has spread.

Top 5 questions-

Based on your opinion, and tests results, what is my survival rate?

If I am in remission (the cancer stops growing), what is the chance that it will come back?

Is my tumor benign or malignant?

Should other members of my family be tested for this type of cancer?

What is my treatment, and how successful do you think it will be?

Additional questions you may consider asking-

How often should I be checked for further spread of my cancer?

What are the risks verses benefits of surgical treatment or chemotherapy?

What can I do to prevent the spread of this cancer?

Carpal Tunnel Syndrome

Carpal tunnel syndrome is caused by compression (pinching) of the median nerve at the wrist. It causes numbness and tingling of the hands and fingers and pain in the wrist and hands. It can happen on one or both wrists. The pain can extend up the arm but usually does not go above the elbow. People with carpal tunnel syndrome also complain of their hands falling asleep. It is often caused by repetitive movements of the wrists but sometimes it can happen spontaneously (for no reason). For mild carpal tunnel syndrome treatment includes wrist braces and over the counter or prescription medications for pain and inflammation as well as avoiding repetitive wrist movements. Moderate or severe carpal tunnel syndrome can sometimes require surgery to release the pressure off of the nerve in the wrist.

Top 5 questions-

Are there non-surgical treatments available?

Can carpal tunnel syndrome happen again after treatment?

How soon after surgery can I return to my normal activities?

Should I wear the braces while asleep?

What can happen if I choose to not have the surgery?

Additional questions you may consider asking-

Are there any blood tests I should have?

Are there any special exercises I can do to make the symptoms go away?

What are the benefits/risks of having both wrists corrected by surgery at once verses one at a time?

Celiac Disease

Celiac disease (also known as Celiac Sprue, or Non-Tropical Sprue) is a condition that damages your small intestines so they can't break down and absorb food properly. The exact cause is unknown, but it is thought to be caused by lack of immunity. Celiac disease causes your body to react badly to gluten or gliadin from grain. Gluten is a protein that is found in wheat. If left untreated, Celiac disease can be serious. Symptoms include diarrhea, abdominal (belly) pain, anemia, bruising, and a rash. Treatment includes a gluten-free diet, certain vitamins, and sometimes medications. In severe cases, hospitalization is sometimes necessary.

Top 5 questions-

Can you please explain to me what a gluten-free diet is?

Should I see a nutritionist?

Should other members of my family be tested for Celiac disease?

What are the results of my endoscopy biopsy and other tests?

What is the purpose of the stool test you are ordering?

Additional questions you may consider asking-

Do I need to see a specialist (gastroenterologist)?

What additional tests do I need and how do I do them?

What are the long-term risks of having this Celiac disease?

What is the purpose of the vitamins you are prescribing?

Cellulitis

Cellulitis is an infection of the skin. It usually begins as a small area of swelling then becomes red and tender. As the red area begins to enlarge, you might develop a fever or swollen lymph nodes (swollen glands) near the area of infected skin. Cellulitis can happen anywhere on the body, but the leg is the most common site, followed by the arm, and then the head and neck. People with obesity (being overweight) can sometimes develop cellulitis in the abdominal (belly) area. Sometimes cellulitis appears in areas where the skin is broken open, but often cellulitis happens where there has been no break in the skin at all. It is treated with antibiotics.

Top 5 questions-

Can my cellulitis lead to other medical conditions?

Is my cellulitis contagious (can be passed to someone else)?

Is there anything I can do to prevent this from happening again?

What, in your opinion, is the cause of my cellulitis?

Why is it necessary to elevate my legs above my heart?

Additional questions you may consider asking-

Do I need any special tests to find the cause of my cellulitis?

How long do you think it will take for the redness and pain to go away?

Is my cellulitis dangerous?

Now that I have had this once, am I at risk for this to happen again?

Will a diuretic (water pill) help eliminate the swelling and make the infection go away faster?

Cerumen Impaction (Ear Wax Blockage)

Cerumen impaction is blockage of the outer ear by tightly packed cerumen (ear wax). Cerumen is the natural ear wax that is made within the ear canal. It helps clean out dead skin cells and prevents dirt and water from entering your inner ear. Cerumen can also protect your ear from infections. Cerumen impaction happens when the ear wax builds up and gets stuck in the ear canal. It can be caused by excessive cleaning of the ears with Q-tips, hearing aid use, or happen spontaneously (for no reason). Cerumen impaction can result in pain and hearing loss.

Top 5 questions-

Are there any ear drops I can use to get rid of the cerumen?

Can you please explain to me how an ear lavage is performed?

I wear a hearing aid. What can I do to prevent a cerumen impaction?

Is there anything I can do to prevent a further increase of wax in my ears?

What is the correct way to clean my ear?

Additional questions you may consider asking-

After the ear lavage, what signs should I look for that there is a complication from the lavage?

Are there any ear drops I can use to prevent another cerumen impaction?

Can I do an ear lavage at home?

How often should I get an ear lavage?

I feel dizziness and have a headache at times. Is this related to my cerumen impaction?

Chest Pain

There are many causes of chest pain. Certain things can trigger your chest pain such as eating a spicy meal, acid reflux, anxiety, lung problems, nerve problems, and several other medical conditions. Chest pain can be nothing more than a simple annoyance, but can be as dangerous as a heart attack. You may not know what is causing your chest pain until you visit your doctor, go to the hospital, or have a variety of tests. If you think the chest pain may be serious it is important to go directly to the emergency room to determine the cause of your pain.

Top 5 questions-

Could my chest pain be related to more than one medical condition?

If I experience this chest pain again, what should I do first?

Is this chest pain related to my heart?

What tests are necessary to determine the cause of my chest pain?

What type of chest pain means it is a cardiac (heart) condition?

Additional questions you may consider asking-

Are over the counter medications safe to use for chest pain?

How does acid reflux cause chest pain?

How does anxiety cause chest pain?

If the chest pain goes away on its own, do I still need to make an appointment to see a doctor?

What type of chest pain means it might be a pulmonary (lung) condition?

Chicken Pox (Varicella)

Chicken pox is a common illness that causes a rash and red spots or blisters (pox) all over the body. It is common in children, and most people will get chicken pox at some point in their lives if they don't have the vaccine. After you have had chicken pox, you are not likely to get it again, but the virus stays in your body long after you get over the illness. If the virus becomes active again, it can cause shingles (this usually happens in older adults). Chicken pox can spread easily by a person with the illness sneezing or coughing on you. You can also get it if you touch the fluid from a chicken pox blister. A person who has chicken pox can spread the virus about 2 to 3 days before the rash appears.

Top 5 questions-

How long will I be contagious?

What are the signs that a blister has become infected?

What can I do for the itching?

What is the best way to prevent me from giving this to someone else?

Will anti-viral medications shorten the time that I have this illness?

Additional questions you may consider asking-

Are there any over the counter creams or treatments to help the itching?

Is there a vaccine that can prevent shingles from happening later in life?

Should I avoid contact with pregnant women?

What is my risk of getting shingles later in life?

Will the blisters leave a permanent scar, and if so, how can I prevent that?

Chronic Kidney Disease

Healthy kidneys remove waste from the blood, then that waste leaves your body in the urine. When the kidneys are damaged, they cannot remove waste from the blood as well as they should. This is called chronic kidney disease. The most common causes of this condition are high blood pressure, diabetes and heart disease. Chronic kidney disease can lead to kidney failure (the kidneys completely not working), but early treatment can slow or prevent this. Most people don't have any symptoms early in the disease, but once it gets worse the symptoms can include feeling tired, weak, or swelling of the legs. Even with treatment, chronic kidney disease can get worse over time and the kidneys can stop working. If this happens, waste builds up in the body and acts like a poison. If the kidneys stop working, then dialysis (a machine that filters waste out of the blood) is necessary.

Top 5 questions-

How often should I have my urine and blood checked?

What dietary changes should I make?

What is my risk of needing dialysis now or in the future?

What is my target number for my blood pressure?

What medications should I avoid since I have kidney disease?

Additional questions you may consider asking-

Are there any other organs affected by my kidney disease?

Should I have other family members tested for kidney disease?

Why do I need to limit protein in my diet?

Chronic Obstructive Pulmonary Disease (COPD)

The term chronic obstructive pulmonary disease (COPD) describes two conditions - chronic bronchitis and emphysema. If you have either of these conditions you are classified as having COPD. These conditions are caused by restriction of air flow and generally present with difficulty breathing. Tobacco smoking is the most common activity that leads to both of these conditions. These two conditions have many similarities, but there are significant differences in terms of how they are treated.

Top 5 questions-

Do I have chronic bronchitis or emphysema?

Do I need any tests to confirm the diagnosis?

How often should I get pulmonary function tests to monitor COPD?

How severe is my COPD?

What can I do reduce the flare-ups of COPD?

Additional questions you may consider asking-

Do I need home oxygen?

Do I need to change any of my daily activities because of COPD?

How often can I use a rescue inhaler?

Should I see a lung specialist (pulmonologist)?

What can I do to keep the airways from building up mucus?

Which immunizations/vaccines should I get and how often?

Cirrhosis

Cirrhosis is a long-term condition where normal liver cells are damaged and begin to die. This causes the liver to not function as it should. In the early stages of cirrhosis you may not know it is happening. Eventually, cirrhosis can cause complete liver failure where the liver completely stops working. Cirrhosis can be caused by drinking too much alcohol, hepatitis, certain diseases, medications, and changes in the area around the liver itself causing blockage of the biliary tract (the tube the carries bile). Cirrhosis can eventually lead to symptoms like ascites (fluid build up in the belly) and jaundice (yellowing of the skin). Cirrhosis is a serious medical condition that will require a great deal of attention by your doctor.

Top 5 questions-

Am I contagious (can pass this to someone else)?

If I stop drinking alcohol will my cirrhosis get better?

What additional tests do I need and how do I do them?

What changes should I make to my diet or lifestyle?

What medications (that filter through the liver) should I avoid?

Additional questions you may consider asking-

Am I a candidate for a liver transplant?

Do I need to see a specialist (gastroenterologist)?

Should I remove all salt from my diet?

Will my ascites and jaundice ever go away with treatment?

Colorectal Polyps

Colorectal polyps are small lumps of tissue in the lining of the colon and rectum (the colon and rectum are part of the intestines). In most cases they are benign (not cancerous). One type of polyp, adenomatous polyp, has the potential to develop into cancer over time. Sometimes polyps will cause bleeding from the rectum or pain in the abdomen but in most cases they cause no symptoms and are only discovered during a routine colonoscopy. Your doctor can also check your stool for blood to screen you for polyps. Increased age, a high fat diet, and family history of polyps make you at increased risk to develop polyps.

Top 5 questions-

Do I need a colonoscopy, CAT scan or other test to make the diagnosis?

How was my polyp found, what did it show, and what does that mean?

What are the advantages and disadvantages of performing a virtual colonoscopy (swallowing a camera the size of a pill that takes pictures of your colon)?

What changes to my diet will decrease my risk of developing more colorectal polyps?

What is the chance I can develop cancer from my polyp?

Additional questions you may consider asking-

At what age do I need my first routine colonoscopy?

How often should I have a colonoscopy?

Should other family members be tested for polyps?

Will I develop more polyps?

Congestive Heart Failure (CHF)

Congestive heart failure (CHF) is when the heart doesn't pump blood as well as it should. The symptoms of CHF are usually shortness of breath, chest pain, weight gain, or a hard time breathing when laying down flat. This condition can also have other less common symptoms like tiredness, fatigue, or poor appetite. CHF may happen when the heart's ability to pump blood becomes impaired (systolic heart failure) or when the heart muscles become too stiff and cannot relax (diastolic heart failure). CHF can be caused by high blood pressure, heart attacks, and certain infections. CHF often goes through periods when the symptoms get worse and the person needs to go to the hospital. These periods are called exacerbations, and are one of the most common causes of hospitalization.

Top 5 questions-

What can happen to me (what are my risks) now that I have CHF?

What is my ejection fraction and what does that mean (tells how well the heart is pumping. Normal ejection fraction is around 50%)?

What is the cause of my congestive heart failure? How severe is it?

What lifestyle and diet changes do you recommend?

What tests do I need to know more about my CHF?

Additional questions you may consider asking-

Do I need a heart transplant (sometimes necessary in severe CHF)?

How do the medications I am taking for congestive heart failure work?

How often should I check my weight and when should I contact you?

What can I do to prevent CHF from getting worse?

Conjunctivitis (Pink Eye)

Conjunctivitis, also known as pink eye, is an inflammation of the conjunctiva (lining that covers the inner surface of the eyelids). It is a common condition caused by viral or bacterial infections, allergens, or foreign bodies in the eye.

Top 5 questions-

Can I go to work with pink eye? If not, how long do I need to be out?

How can I prevent pink eye from happening in the future?

I wear contact lenses. Can I wear them when I have pink eye?

Is pink eye contagious (can be passed to another person)?

What is causing my pink eye?

Additional questions you may consider asking-

Are there certain times of the year I am more likely to get pink eye?

Do I need to see a specialist (ophthalmologist, allergist)?

Do you recommend any changes to my home or work environment to prevent this from happening again?

How long should I expect my pink eye to last?

Is this likely to happen again?

What are the possible risks from having pink eye?

Will I benefit from wearing glasses instead of contacts?

Constipation

Constipation can mean different things to different people. It can be infrequent stools or very hard stools or a combination of both. People can have temporary constipation from traveling or changes in their diet. Some people will suffer from chronic constipation. Depending on the severity or type of constipation the treatment can include stool softener medications, laxatives, or a combination of both. Often dietary changes are necessary such as increasing fiber in your diet. Medically, constipation is usually defined as fewer than three bowel movements a week. Constipation can sometimes be associated with rectal pain, abdominal (belly) pain, and bloating.

Top 5 questions-

Are there changes in my diet I can make to avoid constipation?

Do I need a colonoscopy or an x-ray?

How long can I safely wait between bowel movements?

Should I be taking a laxative every day?

Will exercise help?

Additional questions you may consider asking-

Are there special times of the day I should be going to the bathroom?

What can I do if I over treat my constipation and get diarrhea?

What if I push really hard and see blood; is that dangerous?

Cough

Cough is a very common symptom. Doctors usually classify a cough by its duration: an acute cough existing for less than three weeks, sub-acute cough from three to eight weeks, and chronic cough lasting more than eight weeks. An acute cough is most commonly caused by a respiratory tract infection such as bronchitis or pneumonia or it may be caused by a flare-up of another medical condition (chronic obstructive pulmonary disease, asthma, congestive heart failure). An important issue to understand is that there are a variety of medical conditions including certain medications and acid reflux that can trigger a cough. A cough may be productive of phlegm/sputum or it may be non-productive (dry cough).

Top 5 questions-

Do I need a chest x-ray, CAT scan, or pulmonary function tests?

How long should I expect this cough to last?

What are the possible risks from having a cough?

What is the cause of my cough? Is it contagious (can pass to someone)?

What over the counter treatments are available for my cough?

Additional questions you may consider asking-

Can medications I take for other conditions cause a cough?

How does smoking cause my cough?

If my sputum changes from white to yellow, does that mean I have a bacterial infection?

What does it mean if I see blood in my sputum (hemoptysis)?

Cushing's Syndrome

This is a medical condition caused by high levels of a steroid hormone called cortisol. This hormone is produced by an organ called the adrenal gland. Many people who take steroid hormones for treatment of other conditions can develop Cushing's syndrome. In other cases, this condition is caused by extra production of cortisol by the adrenal gland. Cushing's syndrome presents with weight gain, accumulation of fat on the back of the neck, high blood pressure and a rounded face.

Top 5 questions-

Do I need to see a specialist (endocrinologist)?

How is the diagnosis of Cushing's syndrome made?

What are my treatment choices for Cushing's syndrome?

What is the cause of my Cushing's syndrome?

Which additional tests do you recommend at this time?

Additional questions you may consider asking-

How will my response to treatment be monitored?

I take steroid medications. What can I do to prevent Cushing's syndrome?

Is Cushing's syndrome likely to last my whole life?

Should other people in my family be tested for Cushing's syndrome?

What are the risks of having Cushing's syndrome?

What kind of response can I expect from the treatment of this condition?

Delirium

Delirium is sudden changes in the way a person acts or behaves. People who are delirious are often confused, agitated or have a hard time focusing. A number of medical problems (infections, deafness, and stroke) and certain medications can cause delirium. Elderly people are at higher risk for having delirium, especially when they are in an environment that is different from their routine (like being hospitalized). People who are delirious often do not know they are having this problem and may need other people to bring it to their attention and help them get care. People with delirium can seem like they have dementia (like Alzheimer's disease), but delirium comes and goes, so the person may seem normal sometimes in the day, but start acting differently over a couple of hours. Delirium can sometimes get worse at night.

Top 5 questions-

Are there tests that need to be done to find the cause of the delirium?

Is this delirium or dementia, and what is the difference?

What are the risks of having delirium?

What can be done to keep a delirious person safe when they are confused?

What is causing the delirium? What can be done to make it go away?

Additional questions you may consider asking-

Are there medications that can cause delirium?

How long will the delirium last?

Is delirium an early sign of dementia?

Is delirium likely to happen again?

Dementia

Dementia is not one single disease but rather a group of symptoms that include problems with reasoning, judgment, and memory that interfere with daily functioning. Memory loss is commonly present in people with dementia, but memory loss by itself does not make the diagnosis of dementia. There are many types of dementia, with Alzheimer's dementia being the most common type. Some other types include vascular dementia, Lewy body dementia and Parkinson's dementia. People themselves may or may not be able to recognize their dementia and may need family members to help them get the care they need.

Top 5 questions-

Can the dementia be treated so it goes away, or will it continue to get worse?

Is there a way to stop it from getting worse, or to slow it down?

What are the goals for treatment of dementia?

What can I expect as the dementia gets worse?

What type of dementia does my family member have?

Additional questions you may consider asking-

Are people with dementia allowed to drive?

Are there other tests that need to be done?

Can a person with dementia be safely taken care of at home?

Should other family members be tested for dementia?

Should we see a specialist (neurologist or a geriatrician)?

What are the risks of having dementia?

What resources are available for family members who take care of people with dementia?

Which medications should someone with dementia not take?

Will things like crossword puzzles or changes to the environment (such as reducing noise) stop the dementia from getting worse?

Depression

Depression is a term used to describe many different medical conditions. General depression is the most common form, is mild, and affects millions of people. Symptoms can include insomnia, sad feelings, loss of energy and fatigue. Within this group of diseases are also atypical depression (depression without the usual symptoms), postpartum depression (after delivery of a child), bipolar depression (involving mood swings), seasonal depression, and psychotic depression. Doctors agree that depression comes from a chemical imbalance in the brain but it is also caused by an event such as the loss of a loved one, major life change, or other life crisis. Treatments that are prescribed include psychotherapy, counseling, biofeedback and/or medications. Most medications prescribed for depression are individualized and based on the symptoms. Many doctors prescribe medications called "selective serotonin receptor inhibitors" (SSRIs for short). These medications can correct the chemical imbalance in the brain and can cause symptoms to get better or go away.

Top 5 questions-

Are there treatments that don't involve medications?

Could my depression be caused by another illness?

Should I see a psychiatrist or counselor?

What do I do if I feel like I want to hurt myself of someone else?

Will I always suffer from depression?

Additional questions you may consider asking-

How long after I start taking medicines will I see a change in symptoms?

How long will I need to take my medications?

Dermatitis

Dermatitis is inflammation of the skin. There are different types of dermatitis such as contact dermatitis, atopic dermatitis (eczema), seborrhea dermatitis, dyshydrotic dermatitis, and nummular dermatitis. Most dermatitis conditions are limited to the skin, but some can be a symptom of other medical conditions such as obesity (being overweight), lupus, or Parkinson's disease. Contact dermatitis is caused by contact between the skin and certain substances (soaps, cleaning agents) or allergies (poison ivy, latex). Atopic dermatitis is a chronic skin condition that runs in the family. Seborrhea dermatitis is seen in oily areas of the skin such as the scalp (dandruff) and face.

Top 5 questions-

Is the type of dermatitis I have likely to last my whole life?

Should I be tested for other medical conditions?

What are the possible causes of my dermatitis?

What are the risks of having dermatitis?

Which food, medications, soaps, detergents or jewelry should I avoid?

Additional questions you may consider asking-

Do you recommend any herbal medicines for dermatitis?

Do you recommend any over the counter skin treatments?

Should I change my work or home environment in any way?

Should I have any specialized testing such as a patch test?

Should I wear an allergy bracelet or carry an anaphylaxis kit?

Diabetes

Diabetes is a medical condition that involves high blood glucose (sugar) in the body. Diabetes is caused by too little insulin production from the pancreas or no insulin production at all. Insulin helps your body break down sugar, and without insulin, glucose (sugar) levels in your body can get very high. Diabetes can happen at any age. Many people with diabetes don't have any symptoms, however some people may have a dry mouth, drink a lot of water, and urinate a lot. It is treated with oral medications, insulin, or a combination of both depending on the severity of the disease. It is important to treat diabetes because if your sugar level gets too high, it can cause you to go into a coma, and after years of high sugar levels you can develop many problems with your kidneys, eyes, and heart.

Top 5 questions-

Can my diabetes be better controlled and will I have fewer problems if I start insulin early?

Do I have Type I diabetes or Type II diabetes?
- What does this mean to me and my family?

Should I see a specialist (endocrinologist)?

What do I do if my blood sugar is too high or too low?

What is my hemoglobin A1C level (this test shows the average of all blood sugar levels over a 3 month period of time)?

Additional questions you may consider asking-

How often should I check my blood sugar levels at home?

How often should I get a routine diabetic eye examination?

If I loose weight, will that help lower my blood sugar levels?

Is there anything I should do before or after strenuous exercise?

Should other family members be tested for diabetes?

What are my diabetic ABC's (A = A1C, B= blood pressure, C=cholesterol)? What are my target numbers for my diabetic ABC's?

What can I do to prevent leg ulcers?

What foods should I avoid?

What is a normal range for my blood sugar levels without eating and after eating?

What is my cholesterol level and blood pressure level and what are the recommended levels for a person with diabetes?

What is the best way to care for my feet?

Would I benefit from seeing a dietitian?

Diarrhea

Diarrhea is loose and watery stools. It is a common symptom that usually goes away on its own after a couple days. Sometimes diarrhea can lead to a lot of fluid loss from the body which can cause dehydration. Diarrhea can be caused by infections, intolerance to food items (such as lactose intolerance or gluten sensitivity), a side effect of medications, or by irritable bowel syndrome, inflammatory bowel disease or colon cancer.

Top 5 questions-

Can I take over the counter medications for my diarrhea?

How can I prevent future episodes of diarrhea?

I have been having diarrhea for the last 2-3 months. Which tests do you recommend to figure out what is wrong?

I am having loose stools lately. Does that mean I have an infection?

What are the signs of dehydration and how can I prevent it?

Additional questions you may consider asking-

Are any of the medications I am taking causing diarrhea?

How do I maintain a food diary?

I am having diarrhea alternating with constipation. What does that mean?

I have loose stools mixed with blood. What does that mean?

I started getting diarrhea since I returned from a visit to a foreign country. Which infections should I be checked for?

What are the risks of having diarrhea?

Diverticulosis

The condition of having diverticula (large pouches) in the large intestine or colon is called diverticulosis. This is a common condition that affects about 1 in 10 Americans and it involves the outpouching of the lining of the large intestine through weak spots. Most people with diverticulosis do not have any symptoms, however, it can present with symptoms such as stomach pain or discomfort or bleeding from the rectum, especially when the diverticula are inflamed (*diverticulitis*). This condition is commonly diagnosed by tests such as a CAT scan or colonoscopy.

Top 5 questions-

How can I prevent *diverticulitis* (inflammation of the diverticula)?

How does diverticulosis develop?

What are the risks of having diverticulosis, and how can I prevent it?

What type of diet do you recommend for people who have diverticulosis?

Which conditions increase the risk of developing diverticulosis?

Additional questions you may consider asking-

Can diverticulosis cause cancer?

I was found to have diverticulosis on a CAT scan. What should be the next step in my management?

Should I avoid seeds and nuts if I have diverticulosis?

Since constipation increases my chance of developing diverticulosis, what can I do to prevent constipation?

Dizziness

The word dizziness can describe a variety of sensations such as feeling faint or lightheaded, a spinning sensation, or feeling unsteady. Sensations of spinning are specifically referred to as vertigo. Dizziness that is accompanied by a sudden loss of consciousness with a rapid recovery is called syncope. Dizziness is a common reason for a doctor's visit. Many medical conditions can cause dizziness: some common conditions include ear problems, rapid changes in position, a drop in blood pressure, stress and anxiety, heart irregularities, and severe pain. In addition, certain medications can cause dizziness.

Top 5 questions-

How long is my dizziness likely to last?

What are the non-medicine treatments for dizziness?

Which restrictions should I follow (driving or working with machinery)?

Which tests do you recommend to further evaluate my dizziness?

Why do I get dizzy?

Additional questions you may consider asking-

Are there medications that will make my dizziness go away?

Do any of the medications I take cause dizziness?

I get dizzy when I don't eat. What does that mean?

I get dizzy when I stand up. What does that mean?

What things do you suggest to avoid future dizziness episodes?

Dysmenorrhea (Painful Menstrual Cramps)

Dysmenorrhea is a condition of crampy pain in the lower part of the stomach, thighs or lower back around the time of menstruation. In some cases the pain may be combined with other symptoms such as dizziness, fatigue or nausea. Dysmenorrhea, for some people, can be quite disabling. Conditions such as endometriosis, fibroids, and pelvic inflammatory disease may cause dysmenorrhea, but in most cases the exact cause of dysmenorrhea is not found. Dysmenorrhea symptoms usually improve with advancing age.

Top 5 questions-

I get menstrual cramps, does that mean I have dysmenorrhea?

I get severe menstrual cramps with each menstrual cycle. Can I do anything to prevent these frequent painful episodes?

What are some of the non-medicine treatments for dysmenorrhea?

What tests do you recommend to further evaluate my dysmenorrhea?

Will birth control pills or an intrauterine device (IUD) help my symptoms?

Additional questions you may consider asking-

Are there any herbal medicines that can help my dysmenorrhea?

Do you recommend any exercises to help my dysmenorrhea?

Does dysmenorrhea mean I have cancer?

Does dysmenorrhea reduce fertility (the ability to have children)?

I take over the counter pain medications when I get menstrual cramps. What precautions should I take with these medications?

Dysuria (Painful Urination)

Dysuria is a burning pain that a person feels during or directly after urination. The pain is usually in the area of the urethra (the tube that transports the urine) and not in other areas. Dysuria can be from many causes. The most common reason is a urinary tract infection but it can also be caused by a kidney stone, strictures (scars in the urethra) or from non-medical reasons. A urinalysis is the best way to determine the cause but sometimes an x-ray or blood test is necessary depending on the severity or length of time a person has had dysuria.

Top 5 questions-

If I see blood in my urine and have dysuria, what does that mean?

If the urinalysis is normal, are there other tests (x-ray, blood test) that can find the cause of my dysuria?

Is there anything I can do to prevent dysuria?

What is the cause of my dysuria?

What other symptoms can I look for means there is an infection or a kidney stone?

Additional questions you may consider asking-

Could I have any other medical conditions that are causing my dysuria?

Should I see a specialist (urologist)?

Ear Infections

Ear infections include common medical conditions such as otitis externa (infection of the outer ear), otitis media (infection of the middle ear), and labyrinthitis (infection of the inner ear). Ear infections are much more common in children than in adults. These infections can be acute (usually lasting for a few days) or can become chronic if they last for more than a few weeks or keep coming back.

Top 5 questions-

How long will my symptoms last?

What are the possible risks from having this infection?

What is the cause of my ear infection (virus, bacteria or fungus)?

What treatments do you recommend? Do I need antibiotics?

Which part of the ear is involved in my infection?

Additional questions you may consider asking-

Am I at a high risk for complications from this infection?

Am I likely to spread this infection to people around me?

How can I prevent future ear infections?

Is my ear drum broken (broken ear drums heal by themselves, but you may need to see an otolaryngologist for surgical repair of the ear drum)?

Is there extra fluid (serous otitis media) in my ear (extra fluid increases your chances of getting another ear infection)?

Will I be able to work with this infection?

Ear Pain

Ear pain can be caused by many medical conditions such as ear infections, ear wax, allergies, trauma to the ear (from putting objects in the ear such as pencils, pins) or the eustachian tubes (the tubes that run from the nose to the ears) not working like they should. In many cases ear pain is not caused by the ear itself, but by something called referred pain (sinus pain, tooth pain) that is pain felt in the ear that is actually coming from another source.

Top 5 questions-

Do I need to see an ear specialist (otolaryngologist)?

I have ear drainage. Does that mean I have an infection?

What are the possible risks from having the condition that is causing my ear pain?

What is the cause of my ear pain? Is it infectious or non-infectious?

What medications can I take to treat my ear pain?
- Are any of these medications available over the counter?

Additional questions you may consider asking-

Do I need a pair of earplugs and how do I select the correct earplugs for me?

I get ear pain during flights?
- Is that normal?
- What can I do to prevent that?

I get ear pain when swallowing. What does that mean?

If I don't treat my ear pain, can I get hearing loss?

Endometriosis

In this condition, the normal tissues that line the uterus (referred to as the endometrium) grow outside of uterus. This growth usually happens in the pelvis (the lowest part of belly) but can happen anywhere, and most people with this condition have involvement of more than one site. The exact cause of endometriosis is not known but there are certain risk factors that increase your risk for this condition. Endometriosis presents with dysmenorrhea (pain with menstruation), heavy periods (menorrhagia) or infertility.

Top 5 questions-

How is the diagnosis of endometriosis made?

I get menstrual cramps. Does that mean I have endometriosis?

Is endometriosis a cancerous condition?

What are my treatment choices for endometriosis?

Which parts of my body has endometriosis?

Additional questions you may consider asking-

Does endometriosis always require surgery?

If I have a hysterectomy, will it cure my endometriosis?

What are my risk factors for endometriosis?

What can I do to prevent endometriosis?

What is my risk of getting more endometriosis?

Epistaxis (Nose Bleeds)

Epistaxis is a common medical condition and usually is not related to more serious medical conditions. In most cases your doctor will determine if the epistaxis is caused by any other medical conditions through an examination and possibly a blood test, then will give you suggestions on how to control the bleeding if it happens again. Sometimes nasal sprays to moisturize nasal membranes or control inflammation will be prescribed. If the bleeding cannot stop or has been going on for a long time your doctor might perform a cautery procedure (burning of the blood vessels) or pack the nose with gauze to stop the bleeding. The most common reason for epistaxis is dry nasal membranes.

Top 5 questions-

How long should I wait or what should I do before contacting a doctor?

What can I do at home to prevent this from happening again?

What can I do to stop the bleeding if this happens at home?

What other signs should I be looking for that can show that this is more than just dry nasal membranes?

Will a humidifier running at night help prevent my epistaxis?

Additional questions you may consider asking-

Are there any special tests that can be done to make sure that I don't have a bleeding disorder?

Should I see a specialist (ear nose and throat doctor)?

Will a saline nasal spray before I go to sleep help prevent epistaxis?

Erectile Dysfunction (Impotence)

This is a medical condition defined as not being able to get or keep an erection firm enough for sexual intercourse. This condition is also commonly referred to as impotence or ED. Erectile dysfunction is very common. It can be caused by many different things including medications, high blood pressure, diabetes, smoking, and stress.

Top 5 questions-

Are there any tests to prove I have ED or find out why I have it?

How do I talk to my partner about this?

What are the possible causes of my erectile dysfunction?

Will I be a candidate for treatment with sildenafil (Viagra)?

Will I benefit from psychological counseling? If yes, should I also involve my partner in this activity?

Additional questions you may consider asking-

Are any of the medications I take causing erectile dysfunction?
- If I stop these medications, will the erectile dysfunction improve? If yes, how long will it take to improve?

Have I been tested for common conditions that can cause ED?

How do I choose between sildenafil (Viagra), vardenafil (Levitra) and tadalafil (Cialis): are they all equal in terms of success, side effects and cost?

What lifestyle changes (such as smoking cessation) do you suggest I make to improve my erectile dysfunction?

Fatigue

Fatigue is a symptom, not a medical condition. It can be described as tiredness, lack of energy and motivation, and/or exhaustion. It sometimes can also come with drowsiness. Fatigue is a very common complaint and in many cases is related to things such as stress, lack of sleep or poor nutrition. If correcting these things does not resolve your fatigue then evaluation for other medical conditions will be necessary. Additionally, it is important to remember that some medications can cause fatigue. If fatigue lasts for a long time, and causes you to not be able to carry out your daily activities, then it is called chronic fatigue syndrome.

Top 5 questions-

Do I need any special tests to find the cause of my fatigue?

I always feel tired. Is that normal?

What can be making me feel so tired and unmotivated?

Which medical conditions can cause fatigue?

Will exercise help improve my fatigue?

Additional questions you may consider asking-

Are any of the medications I am taking causing fatigue?

Poor sleep causes fatigue. How can I improve the quality of my sleep?

What are some causes of chronic fatigue syndrome?

What are some of the non-medicine treatments for fatigue?

Fever

Fever is a common symptom and is generally because of an infection. The infection may be from a virus (does not require an antibiotic) or a bacteria (requires an antibiotic). There are a few medical conditions which are not infections that may still cause a fever. Also, some medications can cause a fever. Fever is sometimes combined with chills or shakes along with feeling tired, lack of appetite and difficulty concentrating.

Top 5 questions-

Can I go to work when I have a fever?

I get a fever in the evenings. What does that mean?

What is the cause of my fever?

What tests should I have to find the cause of my fever?

Which medications do you recommend for my fever? Is one better than another?

Additional questions you may consider asking-

Are any of the medications I am taking causing my fever?

Are over the counter medications good for treating fever?

How long do you think my fever will last?

How many tablets of acetaminophen (Tylenol) can I take in one day for my fever?

What things can I do (that doesn't involve medications) to lower my fever?

Fibromyalgia

Fibromyalgia is a medical condition in which multiple joints, muscles and tendons (tissues that connect muscles to bones) hurt and the person usually feels fatigued (tired). Your doctor may identify tender points (places on your body where slight pressure causes pain) in order to make the diagnosis. Fibromyalgia is not a well understood condition, but it is common and happens more in women than men. It is associated with depression and sleep difficulties and it is sometimes difficult to treat.

Top 5 questions-

Do I need to have any tests to confirm the diagnosis of fibromyalgia?

What are some of the risks of having fibromyalgia?

What are my treatment choices for fibromyalgia?

What, in your opinion, is causing my fibromyalgia?

Will the fibromyalgia last my whole life?

Additional questions you may consider asking-

Do I need to see a specialist (rheumatologist) for my fibromyalgia?

Does acupuncture help fibromyalgia?

Does fibromyalgia run in the family?

I also have arthritis in multiple joints. How do I tell the difference between fibromyalgia and arthritis?

Which exercises will help relieve my fibromyalgia pain?

Gallstones

The gallbladder is a small pear shaped organ located on the right side of the belly just below the liver. It holds digestive juices which sometimes harden and form pebble like stones called gallstones. Gallstones are common, but not all people who have gallstones have symptoms from the stones and in many people the stones are only detected by tests (ultrasound or CAT scan) performed for some other reason. Symptoms from gallstones can be stomach pain, nausea and vomiting. Symptoms are usually worse when you eat a fatty meal. Gallstones can lead to inflammation of the gallbladder wall (cholecystitis) and inflammation of the duct (tube) that carries digestive juices from the gallbladder to the intestine (cholangitis).

Top 5 questions-

Can gallstones go away without treatment?

Do I need a surgery for my gallstones?

I have never had any pain and I have gallstones. Is that possible?

What are my risk factors for developing gallstones?

What are the possible risks from having gallstones?

Additional questions you may consider asking-

Can my body function without a gallbladder?

Do I need to avoid fatty meals for my whole life?

What are the different types of gallstones? What type do I have?

What are the possible risks of a gallbladder surgery?

Ganglion Cyst

A ganglion cyst is a gel-like cyst that occurs on the tendon sheath of the top portion of the wrist. It can also occur on the top portion of the ankle. Most ganglions are not painful but sometimes they can cause pain. Ganglions are not dangerous and if they don't bother the person they can be left alone. Sometimes they will break and go away on their own. A common in-office procedure is to aspirate (draw out) the cyst with a large needle to remove the gel. If the cyst returns after aspiration or bothers the person greatly it can be removed surgically.

Top 5 questions-

Can I get more ganglion cysts?

Can I leave it alone and do nothing?

Can you please describe the procedure to aspirate the cyst?

What are the risks or complications of having the cyst aspirated?

Will the cyst get bigger?

Additional questions you may consider asking-

How long will I have to wear the pressure bandage after the aspiration?

Is it necessary to have the cyst surgically removed if the aspiration doesn't work?

What is the chance that the aspiration will not work?

What should I do if I have significant pain and swelling in the area of the pressure bandage after the aspiration?

Gastritis

Gastritis is irritation of the stomach lining. Symptoms often include stomach pain, nausea and vomiting. Gastritis is a common medical condition and can be caused by stress, certain foods, alcohol, medications or Helicobacter pylori infection (bacteria that can live in the stomach and cause an ulcer). Gastritis can be temporary or in some cases it may become chronic and last your whole life.

Top 5 questions-

How can I be checked for a Helicobacter pylori infection?

How long do you think my gastritis will last?

What can cause gastritis or make it worse?

Which foods and medications should I avoid because of my gastritis?

Will over the counter antacids (Mylanta, Rolaids, and Tums) or ranitidine (Zantac) help my symptoms?

Additional questions you may consider asking-

Can I still take an aspirin every day?

Do I need to get any other tests to figure out why I have gastritis?

I get a lot of gas and bloating, do you think it is from my gastritis?

What are my treatment choices for gastritis?

What are the risks of having gastritis?

Gastro-Esophageal Reflux Disorder (GERD)

GERD is sometimes called heartburn. It is caused by the muscles around the opening of the stomach not tightening enough and a small amount of stomach acid going up (refluxing) into the esophagus. GERD causes burning and pain in the chest. It can usually be controlled with over the counter medications or lifestyle changes but sometimes requires prescription medications. The most commonly prescribed medication for this disorder is called omeprazole (Prilosec).

Top 5 questions-

Are there other things I can do to prevent GERD?

Should I be concerned about an ulcer?

What changes in my diet or how I eat can help my symptoms?

What is the best time of the day to take my medication?

Will weight loss help my GERD symptoms?

Additional questions you may consider asking-

Can I take my medicine as needed or does it need to be taken every day?

Do I need to have an endoscopy examination?

What are the symptoms of an ulcer?

Will antacids (Mylanta, Rolaids, Tums) or ranitidine (Zantac) help my symptoms? Can I take these with my omeprazole?

Will raising the head of the bed a few inches help my symptoms?

Gout

Gout (or Gouty Arthritis) is a form of arthritis that happens when a naturally occurring chemical in the body called uric acid becomes too high. The uric acid crystals are very heavy and tend to settle at the lowest part of the body (the big toe). The crystals are glass-like when you look at them through a microscope. This condition can be very painful and causes redness, warmth and swelling of the affected area. The big toe is the most affected joint, but other joints in the body can also be affected. Treatment includes medications for the pain and swelling and sometimes medications to lower the uric acid level.

Top 5 questions-

How much water should I drink per day to prevent gout?

How often should I have my uric acid level checked?

What diet changes should I make to prevent this from happening again?

What is a normal uric acid level and what is my uric acid level?

Why do people suggest that "red meat" be avoided by those that have gout?

Additional questions you may consider asking-

Are there long-term risks from having gout?

Are there long-term risks from medications for gout?

Should I have other family members checked for high uric acid levels?

Should I see an arthritis specialist (rheumatologist)?

Hay Fever (Allergies)

This medical condition can be either seasonal or year-round and usually presents with nasal congestion, sneezing, runny nose, itching or watering eyes and a sensation of mucus draining down the back of the throat (post-nasal drip). The triggers most commonly associated with seasonal allergies include pollens, grasses, and weeds. Year round (perennial) allergies are caused by dust mites, dander, cockroaches, and molds.

Top 5 questions-

Can you give me an allergy medicine that will not cause drowsiness?

Do you recommend I see a specialist (allergist)?

Should I take allergy medications as needed or take them on a daily basis?

What are the possible triggers for my allergies?

What steps can I take to prevent allergy symptoms?

Additional questions you may consider asking-

Am I a candidate for allergy shots?

How can I eliminate dust mites?

How long will it take my treatment to work?

If I have high blood pressure, are nasal decongestants safe?

What should be a target humidity level to avoid allergies?

What steps can I take to keep my home allergen-free?

Will I benefit from special tests such as a patch test?

Head Lice (Pediculosis)

Head lice are parasites that can be found on the head. Infection with head lice is called pediculosis. Anyone who comes in close contact with someone who already has head lice, or even their contaminated clothing are at risk for getting head lice. Close contact with infested clothing, such as hats or coats; or sharing combs or brushes; lying on a bed or couch that has recently been in contact by a person with lice can cause you to get it. Head lice are usually located on the scalp behind the ears and near the neckline. The symptoms are a feeling of something moving in the hair; itching; and sometimes sores on the head. Treatment includes a special shampoo and extensive cleaning of personal items and your living area.

Top 5 questions-

How long will I be contagious (can pass this to someone else)?

If I see nits (eggs) in my hair after treatment, am I still infested?

Should everyone in the house be treated, even if they have no symptoms?

Should I notify my school or work about this?

What if I see signs of head lice a week after treatment?

Additional questions you may consider asking-

Are there any dangers from the treatment for head lice?

Is there any way I can avoid getting this again?

Should I be off from work or school; and for how long?

What is the best way to clean bedding, clothes, combs and other items?

Hemorrhoids

Hemorrhoids (piles) are swollen and painful veins around the area of the anus and lower part of the rectum. These usually develop because of increased pressure on the veins. People can develop hemorrhoids from conditions such as constipation, pregnancy, anal intercourse or obesity (being overweight).

Top 5 questions-

Can I use over the counter medications to treat my hemorrhoids?

I have pain in the anal and rectal area. Is that from hemorrhoids?

What are the risks from having hemorrhoids?

What are the surgical procedures available to treat hemorrhoids?

What can be done to prevent hemorrhoids?

Additional questions you may consider asking-

Do I need to get tests such as a sigmoidoscopy or colonoscopy for my hemorrhoids?

Do I need to see a specialist (surgeon)?

Does anal intercourse increase my risk of hemorrhoids?

How do I prepare a Sitz bath?

Are prescription medications for hemorrhoids more effective than over the counter medications?

Hepatitis

This term means inflammation of the liver. The liver is an essential organ in your body that is involved in food digestion, production of proteins, and removal of toxins from your body. Hepatitis is commonly caused by alcohol, viral infections (such as hepatitis A, hepatitis B, hepatitis C), medications, or in some cases from immune disorders. Some forms of hepatitis may cause permanent liver damage called cirrhosis.

Top 5 questions-

Do I need to avoid certain foods and medications?

How can hepatitis be prevented?

How severe is my hepatitis?

What are the risks of having hepatitis?

What is the cause of my hepatitis?

Additional questions you may consider asking-

Are my family members at high risk for getting hepatitis from me?

How are infections that cause hepatitis transmitted (passed from person to person)?

I have been diagnosed with hepatitis from alcohol. Will that resolve if I stop drinking alcohol?

I was started on a vaccine to prevent hepatitis B. What do I do if I missed a dose?

What are the risks of hepatitis treatment?

Herpes Zoster (Shingles)

Herpes zoster (also known as shingles) is an infection caused by a virus called the varicella zoster virus. This is the same virus that also causes chicken pox and it is the reactivation of this virus that leads to shingles. Shingles presents with a painful blistery rash that can affect any area of the body but usually involves the lower part of the chest and upper part of the stomach. In many cases this infection goes away by itself, but some people may require medications to stop the virus from making the rash.

Top 5 questions-

How can I prevent shingles? Should I get a vaccine to prevent it?

I had an episode of shingles. Does that mean my immune system is weak?

Is this infection contagious (can it spread from person to person)?

Should I take medication to make the varicella virus go away faster?

What pain medications do you recommend?

Additional questions you may consider asking-

Can I continue to work while I have shingles?

How long does the pain from shingles usually last?

I have received the vaccine for chicken pox. Can I still get shingles?

I never had chicken pox. Can I still get shingles?

Is herpes zoster the same infection as genital herpes?

What are some of the risks from having shingles?

Hirsutism (Abnormal Hair Growth)

This is a medical condition where women develop thick and dark hair in areas where men typically grow hair such as the face, chest, abdomen (belly) and back. This extra hair growth is caused by increased levels of male hormones (androgens). In many cases the exact cause of hirsutism may not be found, but all women with hirsutism still need to be evaluated by a doctor. This is especially important if hirsutism is combined with a deep voice, acne or increased muscle mass. Polycystic ovarian syndrome (PCOS) is the most common identifiable cause of hirsutism.

Top 5 questions-

A number of my relatives have hirsutism. Do I need to be tested?

How long do I need to be treated for hirsutism?

If I have hirsutism, can it cause infertility?

What are my treatment choices?

What tests should I have to evaluate my hirsutism?

Additional questions you may consider asking-

Can weight loss help improve hirsutism?

I have always had hirsutism and recently my voice has become deep. What does that mean?

I have been told that I have hirsutism from polycystic ovarian syndrome (PCOS). What are some other symptoms of PCOS?

Which over the counter hair removal products do you recommend?

Hyperlipidemia (High Cholesterol)

This is a medical term used to describe increased levels of lipids (fats) such as cholesterol and triglycerides in the blood. This condition usually does not cause any symptoms, but it significantly increases your risk of getting medical conditions such as heart disease, strokes, and kidney disease. There are different forms of cholesterol that are checked when your doctor orders a "lipid panel" (blood test). These include LDL cholesterol (bad cholesterol), HDL cholesterol (good cholesterol), triglycerides, total cholesterol and non-HDL cholesterol. The numbers on this blood test determines the best type of treatment to prescribe.

Top 5 questions-

Do you recommend lifestyle changes (diet modification, exercise, weight loss) alone to improve my lipid panel numbers or should I also start a medication at the same time?

How often should I check a lipid panel?

How much improvement in my lipid panel numbers can I expect with lifestyle changes and how much improvement can I expect from the medication you recommend?

What is the type or class of lipid disorder I have?

What should be my goal for LDL cholesterol, HDL cholesterol, triglyceride, total cholesterol and non-HDL cholesterol?

Additional questions you may consider-

Are my children also at risk for developing high cholesterol? Should they also have a blood test?

Do I need to see a specialist (endocrinologist)?

Do you think nutritional supplements such as fish oil will help improve my lipid panel numbers?

How long should I fast (not eat) prior to having a lipid panel blood test?

If I accidentally drink coffee (or other beverage) prior to a lipid panel blood test should I reschedule the test?

Once I am started on a medication to lower my cholesterol, will I be able to come off that medication or will I be on it my whole life?

Since I have been diagnosed with high cholesterol, do I also need to test other family members (brothers, sisters, parents)?

Taking into account my lipid panel numbers, what is my risk for developing heart disease or stroke?

What are the possible risks of having hyperlipidemia?

Hyperparathyroidism

Hyperparathyroidism is a condition of excess parathyroid hormones (PTH). Parathyroid glands are four small glands located in the lower part of the neck and are primarily responsible for maintaining calcium balance. Hyperparathyroidism is commonly caused by an adenoma (non-cancerous growth), hyperplasia (enlargement of parathyroid glands) or by cancer of the parathyroid gland. It can also develop in response to conditions such as low calcium, vitamin D deficiency or kidney disease. Hyperparathyroidism may present with symptoms such as body aches, feeling unwell, depression or excessive urination. It can lead to osteoporosis (thin bones) and kidney stones.

Top 5 questions-

How does hyperparathyroidism present?

How is hyperparathyroidism treated?

What are the possible risks of having hyperparathyroidism?

What is the cause of my hyperparathyroidism?

What tests do you recommend to evaluate my hyperparathyroidism?

Additional questions you may consider asking-

How can I reduce my risk of making kidney stones?

I am diagnosed with osteoporosis. Should I get my parathyroid hormone checked?

I have high calcium in my blood. Do I have hyperparathyroidism?

Should I reduce the intake of calcium in my diet if I have hyperparathyroidism?

Hypertension (High Blood Pressure)

Blood pressure refers to the pressure that blood applies as it travels through the blood vessels that carry blood from the heart to different parts of the body (arteries). Hypertension is the medical condition of increased blood pressure. Many people have hypertension without knowing they have this condition since high blood pressure may not cause any symptoms by itself. Blood pressure is reported by two numbers - systolic (upper number) and diastolic (lower number). The most common form of hypertension is called essential hypertension because there is no clear cause other than a family history. Secondary hypertension, on the other hand, is due to an identifiable (secondary) cause.

Top 5 questions-

Do I need to have any special tests to find the cause of my high blood pressure?

Do you recommend lifestyle changes (diet modification, exercise, weight loss) alone to reduce my blood pressure or should I also start a medication at the same time?

How often should I check my blood pressure?

What are my blood pressure numbers today (systolic and diastolic)?

What is my target numbers for blood pressure (the numbers you should be at or below every time it is checked)?

Additional questions you may consider asking-

Do I need to have an ambulatory blood pressure test (24 hour blood pressure test)?

Do I need to see a specialist (nephrologist or cardiologist)?

How much improvement in blood pressure can I expect with lifestyle changes and how much improvement can I expect from the medication you recommend?

I am under a lot of stress. Can stress cause high blood pressure?

If I check my blood pressure on my own and it is recorded as high, what should I do?

Is it better to take my medications in the morning or in the evening?

Is it possible to lower my blood pressure enough by lifestyle changes (diet, weight loss) so I don't have to take medications?

Should I have a home blood pressure monitor?

Once I am started on a medication to lower blood pressure, will I be able to come off that medication or will I be on it the rest of my life?

What are the risks of having high blood pressure?

What is my daily sodium (salt) limit?

What is the class of medication that you are recommending for my high blood pressure?

What things should I consider when buying a home blood pressure monitor?

Will I need more than one medication to control my blood pressure?

Infertility

Infertility is not being able to get pregnant after at least one year of trying. Women that are able to get pregnant but have repeat miscarriages are also considered infertile. About 12 percent of women in the United States are infertile. It is not only a female problem. Male factors account for about one-third of infertility. Men can be infertile because of alcohol, certain medicines, smoking, health problems, and age. Women can be infertile because of problems with the uterus, endometriosis, infections, alcohol, smoking, obesity (being overweight), stress and age.

Top 5 questions-

Are there any medical conditions causing my infertility?

Are there any ways of increasing a male's sperm count?

Does the male partner need a semen analysis and how is that performed?

What is the risk of multiple births from infertility medications?

What medications are available to increase a women's fertility and how do they work?

Additional question you may consider asking-

Please explain what a hysterosalpinogram is and how it is performed?

What is artificial insemination and how is it performed?

What is in-vitro fertilization and how is it performed?

Will my medical insurance pay for infertility treatments?

Inflammatory Bowel Disease

The term inflammatory bowel disease includes Crohn's disease and ulcerative colitis. These long standing conditions are characterized by inflammation of different parts of the digestive tract and the exact cause of these conditions is not known. Inflammatory bowel disease may also involve other parts of the body such as the joints or skin, and they increase your risk for colon cancer. Knowing whether you have Crohn's disease or ulcerative colitis is important because the treatment is different for each.

Top 5 questions-

Do I have Crohn's disease or ulcerative colitis?

How is the diagnosis of inflammatory bowel disease (Crohn's disease or ulcerative colitis) made?

Should I avoid certain foods or medications to prevent a flare-up?

What are my treatment choices?

What are the possible risks from having inflammatory bowel disease?

Additional questions you may consider asking-

Are there alternative ways to manage my condition other than traditional medications?

Can Crohn's disease or ulcerative colitis lead to colon cancer?

Can stress make Crohn's disease worse?

Do I need a surgery to manage inflammatory bowel disease?

Do my family members also need to be tested for inflammatory bowel disease?

How does smoking cigarettes impact inflammatory bowel disease?

How frequently should I get a colonoscopy?

Should I see a specialist (gastroenterologist)?

What are the risks of the surgery that you are recommending?

What dietary changes and lifestyle changes should I make?

What is the difference between ulcerative colitis and Crohn's disease?

What is the likelihood that my child will also get inflammatory bowel disease?

What other conditions can mimic inflammatory bowel disease?

Which parts of my intestine are involved with this condition?

Insomnia

Insomnia is lack of sleep or the inability to fall asleep. It is probably one of the most common complaints a person brings to the medical visit. Insomnia can be acute (lasting just a few days) or chronic (happens all the time or most of the time). The most common reasons for insomnia are stress, certain medications, and stimulants such as caffeine and nicotine. Treatments include medications and/or various suggestions by the doctor on better sleep techniques.

Top 5 questions-

Are medications for insomnia (sleeping pills) addictive?

Are there any medications I take that could be causing my insomnia?

What food, drinks, and other items should I avoid?
- What is the latest in the day that I can have a caffeine product?

What do you think is the cause of my insomnia?

What things can I do to improve sleep that doesn't involve medicines?

Additional questions you may consider asking-

Could I have any medical conditions that are causing my insomnia?

How much sleep should I have, under normal circumstances?

Is a sleep study necessary?

Will exercise help me sleep better?
- If so, is it better to exercise in the morning or later in the day?

Irritable Bowel Syndrome (IBS)

Irritable bowel syndrome, or IBS, is a medical condition that affects the large intestine. With IBS, your bowels are sensitive to food, stress, and emotions. This causes food to either move too quickly or too slowly through the large intestine. Symptoms include bloating, gas, constipation, or diarrhea. Unlike conditions such as Crohn's disease or ulcerative colitis, IBS does not cause any permanent damage to the large intestine. Symptoms seem to get worse with stress, travel, changes in your normal routine, and not eating enough healthy foods.

Top 5 questions-

Could I be lactose intolerant? How is lactose intolerance diagnosed?

Do I need to have an endoscopy examination? How is that done?

How is IBS diagnosed? Can it be cured?

What are the possible risks of having irritable bowel syndrome?

What dietary changes and lifestyle changes should I make?

Additional questions you may consider asking-

Can IBS lead to colon cancer?

Could my IBS be caused by other medical conditions?

Do you recommend stress management therapy for IBS?

How do I maintain a food diary?

What is the difference between IBS and inflammatory bowel disease?

Will increased water intake help my symptoms?

Kidney Stones (Renal Calculi)

A kidney stone (renal calculi) is a hard, crystalline mineral formed in the kidney that eventually moves into the urinary tract. Kidney stones cause blood in the urine and often severe pain in the low back, flank (side), and groin. About one in every 20 people develops a kidney stone at some point in their life. Dehydration puts a person at risk for kidney stones as well as having a urinary tract infection. Men are more likely to develop kidney stones than women. Some kidney stones may not produce symptoms, but most people with stones complain of a sudden onset of excruciating, cramping pain in their low back, flank and groin. The size of the stone determines whether it can pass on its own (through your urine) or if you will need a procedure to help it pass. Rather than having to undergo treatment, it is best to avoid kidney stones in the first place by always drinking plenty of water.

Top 5 questions-

How much water should I drink per day to prevent kidney stones?

Should I be straining my urine to capture the stone?

What are the risk and/or benefits of having a lithotripsy (ultrasound guided destruction of a kidney stone) verses surgical removal?

What is the best way to prevent forming a stone again?

What is the likelihood that I can pass this stone on my own?

Additional questions you may consider asking-

Are there any changes to my diet I should make to prevent another stone?

If I get a stone again, should I contact you or can I manage it at home?

Should I see a specialist (urologist)?

Leukemia

Leukemia is a cancer that begins in the tissues that form blood (bone marrow). This condition causes your body to make abnormal white blood cells called leukemia cells. These abnormal cells can crowd out normal cells and make it hard for them to work properly. There are many different types of leukemia. Chronic leukemia sometimes has no symptoms but acute leukemia can present with nausea, vomiting, muscle weakness, headaches and seizures. Symptoms common to both types of leukemia are fatigue, sweating at night, swollen glands, weight loss and abdominal (belly) pain. The diagnosis of leukemia usually involves a bone biopsy.

Top 5 questions-

Can my leukemia be cured or just controlled?

How is a bone biopsy done and what bone will be used? Will it hurt?

What are the risks and side effects of my treatment?

What is the survival rate of the type of leukemia I have?

What type of leukemia do I have?

Additional questions you may consider asking-

Am I at higher risk of getting infections or other medical conditions because of my leukemia?

Am I contagious (can pass this to another person)?

Do my family members need to be tested for leukemia?

How long will my treatments last? How often will I need treatment?

Lipoma (Fatty Cyst)

A lipoma is a cyst that is filled with fat that occurs just underneath the skin. Lipomas can occur on any part of the body. Sometimes they can become quite large and sometimes they can occur deeper in the skin tissue. They happen spontaneously (on their own) and will not go away once they have formed. Lipomas are not painful or dangerous. If your doctor is uncertain it is a lipoma, an ultrasound or CAT scan may be ordered to get a better look at the lipoma. Rarely do lipomas need a biopsy and they only need to be removed if they bother the person.

Top 5 questions-

Do I need a biopsy? How is it performed?

Is there any risk in just leaving my lipoma alone?

Is there any chance that this can be something else?

What are the risks verses the benefits of removing my lipoma?

Will it go away on its own?

Additional questions you may consider asking-

Do I need to see a surgeon for the removal?

Since I already have a lipoma, does that mean I am at risk to make more?

What signs should I look for that signals this may be something else or a result of other medical conditions?

Liver Function Tests (LFTs)

Abnormal liver function tests (LFTs for short) is a problem that some people encounter as a part of their doctor's visit. Often a doctor will include LFTs as a part of a routine blood test to see how well the liver is functioning, whether it is safe to take medications that filter through the liver, or if there are any medical conditions involving the liver. Mild elevations in LFTs are common and not particularly dangerous. Significant elevations will require further investigation. Elevations can happen from too much acetaminophen (Tylenol) usage, alcohol, liver or gallbladder conditions, viral infections as well as a variety of other medical conditions.

Top 5 questions-

Am I contagious (can pass this to someone else)?

How dangerous is my elevation in LFTs?

How far above normal are my LFT values?

What medications should I avoid if I have elevated LFTs?

When should I get tested again?

Additional questions you may consider asking-

Are there any symptoms I should look for that signals a more dangerous condition?

Can I continue to take acetaminophen (Tylenol) if needed?

Should I stop all alcohol usage?

What is the purpose of the ultrasound or blood tests you are ordering?

Lyme Disease

Lyme disease is an infection caused by bacteria. Ticks pick up the bacteria from mice, squirrels and deer and can pass it to you when they attach to you. The most common tick that carries the bacteria is the black-legged deer tick. When you are bitten by a deer tick, it will attach itself to your skin. It may take 24 to 28 hours for the bacteria to reach your blood from the tick so the longer it stays on you the higher the chance you can get the bacteria. Deer ticks are commonly found in the Northeastern and North Central United States. Lyme disease can cause several symptoms such as a rash, fever, joint aches, sore throat and weakness. Lyme disease can also cause medical complications such as heart problems, arthritis, and neurological problems.

Top 5 questions-

Can I get this again if I am bitten by another deer tick?

How can I decrease my chances of getting Lyme disease?

How long after treatment will my symptoms go away?

What are the long-term risks of having Lyme disease?

What special tests will you order to make the diagnosis and please explain how these tests are done?

Additional questions you may consider asking-

Is the arthritis, heart problems, or neurological complications from Lyme disease permanent?

Should other family members be tested for Lyme disease even though they don't have symptoms?

What is a "target" rash?

Lupus

Lupus is caused by your immune system attacking your body tissues causing inflammation and damage. Symptoms of lupus include fatigue, joint pain, and a lupus rash (a rash that gets worse after being in the sun). The lupus rash is called a "butterfly" rash because it usually is on the cheeks and looks a like a butterfly. Lupus runs in the family. It is diagnosed with a blood test. In severe cases it can cause multiple joint pain, skin problems, sensitivity to light, swollen glands, swelling of joints, weight loss, and anemia. In mild cases no treatment is necessary, but in severe cases multiple types of treatment may be necessary.

Top 5 questions-

Are there any exercises that can help my symptoms?

Can my lupus be cured, or only controlled?

Is there anything I can do for the rash?

What are the results of my blood tests? How do my numbers compare to normal?

What is Reynaud's phenomenon?

Additional questions you may consider asking-

Do I need to see a specialist (rheumatologist)?

How do I distinguish my lupus pain from other common pain?

How often should I have a blood test to monitor my lupus?

Should my family members be tested for lupus?

What is the long-term risk of having lupus?

Meningitis

This condition is inflammation of an area around the spinal cord (meninges). It is usually caused by an infection. The infection is most often from a virus, but sometimes meningitis can be caused by a bacteria or fungus. Depending on the cause of the infection and how severe the infection is; meningitis can go away by itself in a few weeks or it can turn into a serious medical emergency. The classic symptoms of meningitis are headache, fever and stiff neck. Anyone can get this condition, including newborns. If you live in a community type setting (dormitory, barracks), are pregnant, work with animals, or have a weak immune system, you are at increased risk of getting meningitis. There are vaccines you can get that will protect you from certain viruses that commonly cause meningitis.

Top 5 questions-

Am I contagious (can pass this to someone else)?

Are there any long-term risks from having meningitis?

Do my family members or people that I live with need to take medications to prevent them from getting the same type of meningitis I have?

How did I get my meningitis?

What type of meningitis do I have? Do I need antibiotics?

Additional questions you may consider asking-

What is the difference between bacterial and viral meningitis?

What kind of tests do I need? How are they performed?

When can I expect to feel better?

Menopause

Menopause is defined as the absence of menstrual periods for at least 12 months. Menopause results when the woman's ovaries cease to function. The ovaries are the main source of female hormones (estrogen), which control the development of female body characteristics and they also regulate and maintain the menstrual cycle and protect bones. Women with menopause can develop osteoporosis (thinning of the bones). Some women may experience few or no symptoms of menopause, while others can experience multiple physical and psychological symptoms. Symptoms include irregular vaginal bleeding, hot flashes, changes in emotions and trouble sleeping. Menopause is a natural part of life and in many cases does not require any treatment, but treatment for troublesome symptoms is sometimes necessary.

Top 5 questions-

Are there medications that can help control my hot flashes?

Do I still need to have routine pap smears?

If I begin bleeding again, what does that mean?

Now that I am menopausal, how often should I have a bone density scan?

Should I be taking medications to prevent heart disease and osteoporosis?

Additional questions you may consider asking-

I seem to have a decrease in sexual desire. Is that normal?

Is there anything I can do for my vaginal dryness?

My mother took "hormone" pills for her menopause. Should I take them?

Metabolic Syndrome

Metabolic syndrome consists of a combination of medical problems that, together, increases your risk for heart disease, stroke, and diabetes. This group of medical problems are *high triglycerides* (a type of cholesterol), *low HDL cholesterol* (the 'good' cholesterol), *high blood pressure, high blood sugar* (but not high enough for the diagnosis of diabetes), and extra *fat around your belly*. If you have at least three of these five problems you have metabolic syndrome. People with metabolic syndrome may not have any symptoms but it is important to address each of the medical problems aggressively to prevent the eventual development of heart disease, stroke, or diabetes. Important lifestyle changes to improve metabolic syndrome include losing weight, decreasing the amount of salt in your diet, decreasing your alcohol intake, and increasing your exercise.

Top 5 questions-

Can I take medications to prevent heart disease, stroke, or diabetes?

Does smoking increase my risk even more?

What should my cholesterol, blood pressure, and blood sugar numbers be?

What is my risk of developing heart disease, stroke, or diabetes?

What lifestyle changes must I make to lower my risk?

Additional questions you may consider asking-

Could my metabolic syndrome be from other medical conditions?

If I eliminate at least one or two medical problems from the list, do I still have metabolic syndrome and am I still at risk?

Should I see a nutritionist?

Migraine Headache

A migraine headache is considered to be a "headache syndrome." That means it is a headache unto itself and not caused by a secondary condition. Migraines usually involve nausea, photophobia (sensitivity to light), and can last for hours. Once a patient is established as suffering from migraine headaches they tend to suffer from them throughout their lifetime. Migraines can be brought on by certain triggers and it is important to know what triggers your migraine so you can try to avoid it. There are special medications called triptans that are effective in treating migraines.

Top 5 questions-

At what point do I stop treating the individual migraine headache and start taking a daily medication to prevent the migraine?

Can stress be a trigger for my migraine?

What are some of the triggers that could be causing my migraine?

What is the best way to take my migraine medication? Are over the counter migraine medications available?

What symptoms should I look for that shows this is more than a migraine?

Additional questions you may consider asking-

Do I need to see a specialist (neurologist)?

How many times per day can I take my migraine medicine?

Should I make any lifestyle changes to cause less migraine episodes?

What are some of the risks of taking migraine medications?

What are some treatments for my migraines that don't involve medicines?

Mitral Valve Prolapse

Mitral valve prolapse is when one of your heart valves (the mitral valve - controlling blood flow to your left ventricle) does not close properly. This will usually cause a murmur (a swooshing sound heard when your doctor is listening to the heart) and can also cause a clicking sound. The condition is common, even in healthy people. You can be born with it or develop it later in life or as a result of a childhood illness such as rheumatic fever. It generally does not cause symptoms. You are at risk, though, for an infection of the heart (endocarditis) following certain medical procedures including dental work and may need to take an antibiotic prior to those procedures to prevent an infection.

Top 5 questions-

Do I need an echocardiogram (an ultrasound of heart) to confirm the diagnosis?

Do I need to take antibiotics for a dental cleaning?

Does mitral valve prolapse put me at risk for other heart conditions?

How do I properly take the antibiotics prior to my medical procedure?

What medical procedures require pre-treatment with antibiotics?

Additional questions you may consider asking-

Are heart palpitations related to mitral valve prolapse?

Can I still exercise regularly?

Can it go way on its own?

Do I need a cardiac stress test?

Myocardial Infarction (Heart Attack)

A heart attack (also known as myocardial infarction) is the death of heart muscle due to the sudden blockage of a coronary artery by a blood clot. Coronary arteries are the blood vessels that supply the heart muscles with blood and oxygen. If a coronary artery suddenly becomes blocked, and if blood flow is not restored to the heart muscle within about 30 minutes, irreversible death of the heart muscle will begin. The injury to heart muscles cause chest pain and chest pressure. You may also experience profuse sweating, and/or difficulty breathing. Approximately one million Americans suffer a heart attack each year. While heart attacks can happen at any time, most heart attacks happen between 4:00 A.M. and 10:00 A.M. Smoking cigarettes, high blood pressure, elevated cholesterol, and diabetes can accelerate atherosclerosis (a process where plaque builds up and gradually blocks the arteries) and can lead to a heart attack earlier in life. If you have had a heart attack, you doctor will concentrate on eliminating those risk factors from your life to prevent another heart attack.

Top 5 questions-

How often should I have my cholesterol checked?

Should I be taking an aspirin every day?

What is my risk of having another heart attack?

What is my target blood pressure number?

What is my target cholesterol number?

Additional questions you may consider asking-

How often should I be routinely examined?

How should I take my nitroglycerin if I have chest pain again?

Should I avoid heavy lifting or other strenuous activities?

Should I have routine EKG's (electrocardiogram)?

Should other family members be tested for atherosclerosis?

Should I be seeing a specialist (cardiologist)?

What are the best physical activities for me?

What does the nitroglycerin tablet do when I take it?

When can I return to normal sexual activity?

Will exercise help? What is the appropriate amount of exercise for me?

Why is it necessary to be on a beta-blocker type medication every day?

Why did I have a heart attack?

Nausea and Vomiting

Nausea and vomiting are not medical conditions but symptoms of a medical condition. So many medical conditions can cause nausea and vomiting that they are too numerous to mention in this section. The biggest complication of nausea and vomiting is the loss of body fluids that leads to dehydration. Dehydration is more likely to cause problems in older adults and children.

Top 5 questions-

Am I contagious (can pass this to someone else)?

How will I know I am becoming too dehydrated?

If my symptoms don't go away, how long should I wait before contacting you again?

What, in your opinion, is the cause of my nausea and vomiting?

What is the best fluid I should be drinking to re-hydrate myself?

Additional questions you may consider asking-

Can I take over the counter medications for fever, nausea, vomiting or diarrhea at the same time you are treating my condition?

Do I need any special tests to determine the cause of my nausea and vomiting?

Do I need intravenous fluids (IV)?

I am pregnant. Will any of the medications for nausea harm my child?

If I am not able to hold down my oral medication, is there an alternative way of taking the medication?

Neck Pain

A variety of conditions such as muscle spasms, ligament sprain, arthritis and compression of nerves (pinched nerve) can lead to neck pain. Neck pain may last for a few days (acute) or may last for several weeks (chronic).

Top 5 questions-

Can you recommend any home exercises or physical therapy for my pain?

Do I need any additional tests to diagnose my neck pain?

What activities should I avoid because of my pain?

What is the cause of my neck pain? Is it a pinched nerve?

Which medicines do you recommend, and are they available over the counter?

Additional questions you may consider asking-

Am I likely to get neck pain again?

Can I apply heat or ice to my painful areas?

Do you recommend using a neck collar?

How long do you think my neck pain will last?

If my neck pain gets worse when I start exercise then what should I do?

Is my neck pain likely to get worse with time?

What can I do to prevent my neck pain from getting worse?

Obesity

One in every three people in the United States is obese. Doctors diagnose obesity using a calculation called a body mass index (BMI). This calculation uses your height and weight to determine your body mass. The definition of obesity is a BMI greater than 30. The risk of obesity is great and includes medical conditions such as heart disease, diabetes, high blood pressure, high cholesterol, stroke, congestive heart failure, gallstones, gout, arthritis and sleep apnea. Because obesity can lead to so many medical conditions it is very important to keep your weight in a normal range.

Top 5 questions-

How much weight loss per week or month is considered safe?

Is a medical condition causing my obesity?

What are the risks and benefits of surgery, medications, and dieting? Which do you recommend?

What is my BMI? What is a normal BMI?

What is my risk of developing other medical conditions from my obesity?

Additional questions you may consider asking-

Does it matter where the body fat is located (belly verses all over)?

How much exercise is appropriate for me?

Should I see a dietician?

Will you help me choose a safe weight loss program and monitor my progress?

Osteoporosis

Osteoporosis is a decrease in the density of bone which then decreases its strength and results in fragile bones. Bones that are affected by osteoporosis can break with minor injury that normally wouldn't cause a bone to break. The break (fracture) can either be a crack in the bone or collapsing of the bone (as in a compression fracture of the spine). The spine, hips, ribs, and wrists are common areas of bone fractures from osteoporosis although osteoporosis-related fractures can happen in almost any bone. There are several risk factors for developing osteoporosis; female gender, Caucasian or Asian race, small body frame, family history, smoking, alcohol consumption, lack of exercise, or a diet low in calcium. Treatment is aimed at preventing further weakening of the bones.

Top 5 questions-

How much calcium should I be taking per day?

Should I be taking a bisphosphonate medication (a medication to stop the progression of osteoporosis)?

What can I do to prevent a fracture?

What is my risk of a fracture?

What is the best source of calcium in my diet?

Additional questions you may consider asking-

How often should I have a bone density scan?

How can I decrease my risk of falls and fractures?

Why is vitamin D important?

Will my bones re-gain strength with treatment?

Palpitations

Palpitations are sensations of irregular or forceful beating of the heart. Some people with palpitations have no heart disease and the reason for their palpitations can be unknown. Often palpitations are caused by something as simple as too much caffeine, nicotine, or other stimulants. Palpitations can also be the result of abnormal heart rhythms (arrhythmias). An arrhythmia refers to heartbeats that are too slow, too rapid, or irregular. Many heart arrhythmias require special treatment so your doctor will probably want to perform a complete evaluation of your palpitations before telling you the exact cause. Many palpitations require no specific treatment at all. Others will lead to a variety of treatments from oral medications to cardiac procedures.

Top 5 questions-

Are my palpitations dangerous?

Do I need a cardiac stress test? Do I need a Holter monitor (a heart monitor worn for 24 hours)?

If my palpitations are associated with chest pain, what does that mean?

What, in your opinion, is the cause of my palpitations?

Will drinking decaffeinated drinks or quitting smoking help?

Additional questions you may consider asking-

Can I continue exercising with palpitations?

Do my palpitations put me at risk for heart disease?

What were the results of my EKG (electrocardiogram)?

Will I need to be on these medications for the rest of my life?

Pancreatitis

Pancreatitis is inflammation of the pancreas. The pancreas is a small organ near the stomach that helps digest food and makes insulin. Pancreatitis may start suddenly (acute pancreatitis) or it may last for months to years (chronic pancreatitis). Symptoms include severe pain in the belly, nausea, and vomiting. Conditions such as alcohol use, gallstones or high triglycerides (a type of cholesterol) can cause irritation of the pancreas. People with acute pancreatitis need to be hospitalized whereas people with chronic pancreatitis are generally treated outside of the hospital.

Top 5 questions-

Am I likely to get pancreatitis again?

How is my pancreatitis diagnosed?

What are the possible risks of having pancreatitis?

Which pain medications do you recommend for my pancreatitis?

Why did I get pancreatitis?

Additional questions you may consider asking-

Are there any alternative treatments (other than pain medications) that I can do for the pain of chronic pancreatitis?

Do I need to see a specialist (gastroenterologist)?

How long do I need to be in the hospital for the treatment of pancreatitis (those patients who are hospitalized)?

Which diet changes do you recommend to avoid having pancreatitis again?

Parkinson's Disease

Parkinson's disease is a movement disorder that lasts life-long and generally gets worse over time. It may present with symptoms such as tremors, stiffness of the limbs and trunk, slowness of movement and problems with balance. There are a variety of treatment options available for these symptoms. People with Parkinson's disease may also develop memory problems (Parkinson's dementia).

Top 5 questions-

Do tremors and stiff limbs automatically mean I have Parkinson's disease?

Does Parkinson's run in the family? Are my children likely to get it?

How is the diagnosis of Parkinson's disease confirmed?

What can be done to prevent the progression of Parkinson's disease?

Which medications do you recommend, and how do they work?

Additional questions you may consider asking-

Are there any alternative treatments you recommend for my condition?

Can I drive with Parkinson's disease?

I have been having memory loss. Am I getting Parkinson's dementia?

What are the risks of having Parkinson's disease?

What are your thoughts about stem cell treatment for Parkinson's disease?

What should I tell my family about my Parkinson's disease?

Will I be able to keep my job with Parkinson's disease?

Pharyngitis (Sore Throat)

Pharyngitis is a medical term for sore throat. It can be caused by a variety of infectious agents such as viruses and bacteria. It can also be from drainage of mucus down the back of your throat (post-nasal drip), or irritants such as smoke.

Top 5 questions-

Do I need a throat swab (culture) to confirm the diagnosis?

Do I need antibiotics to treat my sore throat?

Is my pharyngitis contagious (can be spread to people around me)?

What are the possible risks of having pharyngitis?

What is the most likely cause of my pharyngitis?

Additional questions you may consider asking-

Am I allowed to air travel while having pharyngitis?

Am I likely to get this again. If yes, how do I prevent it?

Can my throat infection involve other parts of my body (sinuses, tonsils, heart, kidney, or liver)?

Can you suggest over the counter medications for my pharyngitis?

Do I need to take time off from work because of my pharyngitis?

If my episodes of pharyngitis are recurrent (keep coming back), do I need surgery?

Will a humidifier help prevent getting pharyngitis again?

Plantar Fasciitis

Plantar fasciitis is a common reason for heel pain and is caused by inflammation of a thick structure called the plantar fascia that is located at the bottom of the feet. This condition presents with stabbing heel pain that is usually worse first thing in the morning and when you start walking. In most cases this condition is diagnosed in your doctor's office with just a physical exam, but in some cases special tests such as x-rays may be ordered to look for other possible causes of heel pain such as heel spurs or stress fractures.

Top 5 questions-

Do I need any tests such as x-rays for the diagnosis of this condition?

Do I need to see a specialist (podiatrist) for plantar fasciitis?

Do you recommend foot exercises to improve my plantar fasciitis?

What are some of the long-term risks of having plantar fasciitis?

Will this go away with treatment, and how long until my pain improves?

Additional questions you may consider asking-

Do you recommend night splints for my plantar fasciitis?

I am a marathon runner. What can I do prevent plantar fasciitis?

Should I buy over the counter shoe inserts to improve plantar fasciitis?

Should I change my shoes? Do my high-heels or athletic shoes cause plantar fasciitis?

Should I have a corticosteroid injection in my heel for treatment?

Pneumonia

Pneumonia is inflammation of the lungs that is generally caused by infections. Pneumonia seen in people who are coming from the community is labeled as community acquired pneumonia as opposed to pneumonia that develops in people after being in the hospital labeled as hospital acquired pneumonia. People with pneumonia have fever, cough and breathing difficulties, but these symptoms may not always be present, especially in elderly people. People with milder forms of pneumonia can be treated at home, but those with more severe symptoms are treated in the hospital.

Top 5 questions-

Do I need an x-ray to confirm my pneumonia has gone away and when should I have it?

Do I need to be hospitalized for my pneumonia? Do I need to be started on antibiotics right away?

Is my pneumonia contagious (can be passed to someone else)?

What is the cause of my pneumonia? What is walking pneumonia?

Additional questions you may consider asking-

Can a flu virus cause pneumonia?

How can I prevent future episodes of pneumonia?

If my symptoms don't go away, how long should I wait to see you again?

Is my pneumonia due to Legionnaires' disease?

What are my risk factors for future episodes of pneumonia? How can I modify these risk factors?

Psoriasis

Psoriasis is a skin condition that usually affects the elbows, knees and scalp, but in severe cases can affect the entire body. It presents with thick, dry, scaly patches of skin that sit on a red base and is very itchy. This medical condition is sometimes worse during cold wintery months and can come and go. In some cases it can be gone for many years before returning. The exact cause of psoriasis is unknown. Psoriasis can run in the family. It can involve the nails at times, and about 30% of people with psoriasis will also have joint pain. There are a variety of treatments including creams, oral medication, and light therapy (sitting under intense ultraviolet light for short periods of time).

Top 5 questions-

Am I a candidate for ultraviolet light therapy?

Am I contagious (can pass this to someone else)?

Is my psoriasis curable or can it only be controlled?

What can I do to control the itching?

What can I do to prevent a flare-up of my psoriasis?

Additional questions you may consider asking-

Can my psoriasis only affect my nails and not the skin?

Can stress cause my symptoms to get worse?

Do I need to see a specialist (dermatologist)?

What are the long-term risks of having psoriasis?

What is the likelihood my children will get psoriasis?

Rectal Bleeding

The rectum is the lower part of your large intestine. Rectal bleeding is when there is blood in the stool. Signs of rectal bleeding can be bright red blood in the toilet after a bowel movement, blood on the toilet paper, or very dark colored stool. Many things can cause rectal bleeding, but the most common causes are hemorrhoids and constipation. Rectal bleeding can also be seen in more serious problems like diverticulosis (bleeding pockets in the large intestine) and colon cancer.

Top 5 questions-

How can my rectal bleeding be treated?

I have rectal bleeding but don't have any pain. What does that mean?

What do you think is the most likely cause of my rectal bleeding?

Which tests do I need to figure out the cause of my rectal bleeding?

Will I have more rectal bleeding even after treatment of the condition that caused it?

Additional questions you may consider asking-

Do I need a blood transfusion to replace the blood loss?

How does rectal cancer present?

Should I see a specialist (gastroenterologist) for rectal bleeding?

Should I stop taking aspirin since I have rectal bleeding?

Which dietary changes do you recommend to control rectal bleeding?

Scabies

Scabies is a little animal (mite) that burrows (dig tunnels), lays eggs, and lives under the skin. These mites biting the skin and laying their eggs result in a rash that is called scabies. Most people do not know they have scabies until after the mites have been under the skin for several weeks. The main symptoms are itching and a rash. Scabies spreads quickly and requires treatment with a cream to kill the mites in order for it to go away.

Top 5 questions-

How far should I go back to tell people that I had contact with them and I was infected with scabies?

How is it passed from person to person?

Is my scabies currently contagious (can be passed to other people)?

What is the best way to wash my bedding and my clothes?

Will I need to repeat the treatment after a period of time?

Additional questions you may consider asking-

Do I need to tell my work or school about this?

Do I need to treat other family members, even if they don't have a rash or itching?

I heard you can put clothes and other items in a plastic bag for a week to kill the mites. Is that true?

Is there over the counter or prescription medicine I can use for itching?

What is the correct way to apply the cream?

Scoliosis

Scoliosis is when the spine curves to the side. It usually happens during a growth spurt just before a child becomes a teenager. It sometimes can be the result of other medical conditions such as cerebral palsy or muscular dystrophy, but in most cases the cause is unknown. Most cases of scoliosis are mild and don't require any treatment. Severe cases of scoliosis can be serious and require surgery and/or a back brace to correct the curvature. In come cases you doctor will order an x-ray and ask the radiologist (a specialist that reads x-rays) to measure the exact amount of curvature. The degree of curvature determines if any treatment is necessary. Scoliosis can run in the family. It usually does not cause pain.

Top 5 questions-

Do I need an x-ray?

What are the long-term risks from having scoliosis?

What degree of scoliosis do I have? What degree is considered severe?

When should my scoliosis be checked again?

Will my scoliosis get worse with time?

Additional questions you may consider asking-

Are there any special exercises to correct the curvature?

Do I need to have surgery?

Do I need to see a specialist (orthopedician)?

Do I need to wear a back brace?

Seizures

Seizures happen because of abnormal electrical activity in the brain. They may present with abnormal movements, or changes in behavior. People with recurrent seizures (happening over and over) are considered to have epilepsy. A number of conditions such as low blood sugar or dehydration may provoke a seizure, but often the exact cause of epilepsy is not understood. Seizures are a frightening experience and it is very important to identify the triggers that cause seizures and avoid them if possible.

Top 5 questions-

Am I likely to have seizures for the rest of my life?

Can I drive on my own? If not, when will I be able to drive?

I am on an anti-seizure medication. When can I come off that medication?

What are the possible triggers of my seizures?

What should my family be aware of in case I am about to have a seizure?

Additional questions you may consider asking-

Does epilepsy run in the family?

Is it all right to use generic anti-seizure medication?

What are some of my treatment choices for seizures?

What are the possible risks from having seizures?

What tests do I need to evaluate my seizures? How are they performed?

What work restrictions and precautions should I take if I have a seizure disorder? Are there additional restrictions if I am on a medication?

Sexually Transmitted Diseases (STDs)

Sexually transmitted diseases (STD) are infections transmitted through intimate sexual contact - vaginal intercourse, oral sex or anal sex. Some STDs can also get transmitted through blood transfusions, intravenous needle use, childbirth or breastfeeding. A variety of infections fall under the category of STDs. They include chlamydia, gonorrhea, syphilis, chancroid, herpes simplex 2, hepatitis B and C, human immunodeficiency virus (HIV), human papilloma virus (HPV), mollususm contagiosum, crab louse, and trichomoniasis. Some people with STDs may not even know that they have a STD since infections can remain completely without symptoms and hence practicing safe sex is the key to avoiding transmission of STDs.

Top 5 questions-

Do I need to get tested regularly for STDs even if I don't have symptoms?

How do I prevent future STDs? Are condoms enough protection? Are there vaccines to prevent STDs?

I engaged in unprotected sexual intercourse. Should I be tested for STDs?

If I have a STD, how long should I practice abstinence?

Which STD do I have?

Additional questions you may consider asking-

Can oral sores from a herpes infection be transmitted by oral sex?

Can STDs be transmitted by oral sex, hand shake, or a toilet seat?

Does my sexual partner have to be tested and treated at the same time?

What are the risks from having a STD?

Sinusitis

Sinuses are big air-filled areas in the bones above the eyebrows and below the eyes. The sinuses are connected to the nose, and when you are sick (often with a cold), they can become backed up and fill with fluid. This fluid can get infected and cause sinusitis (sinus infection). Sinuses may also develop long-term irritation called chronic sinusitis that can last longer than 3 months. Conditions such as allergies, polyps, or certain chronic infections are usually the cause of chronic sinusitis.

Top 5 questions-

Do I need antibiotics to treat my sinusitis?

Do you think over the counter decongestants will help my sinusitis?

How long will this episode of sinusitis last? Is it acute or chronic?

What is causing my sinus irritation?

What steps can I take to avoid sinusitis in the future?

Additional questions you may consider asking-

Do I need any tests to see if I have chronic sinusitis?

I have a cough that is not going away. Can this be from sinusitis?

I have been getting frequent episodes of sinusitis. What can be causing these?

If I have high blood pressure, are nasal decongestants safe?

Should I do anything different when having sinusitis?

What are the possible risks of having sinusitis?

Skin Tags

Skin tags are small pieces of extra skin that appear throughout a patient's lifetime. They most commonly occur around the neck but can occur anywhere on the body. Treatment usually involves removing them with a small pair of sterile scissors in the doctor's office (with or without local anesthesia) depending on their size. They are generally removed for cosmetic reasons or because they are bothersome or get in the way of jewelry.

Top 5 questions-

Are there any risks from removing the skin tags?

If I choose not to remove them, what signs should I look for that indicates it is skin cancer or if I should have it checked again by a doctor?

If I remove the skin tags, will they return?

How can I know it is not cancer?

Will removing the skin tags leave a mark or a scar?

Additional questions you may consider asking-

Can I remove the skin tags by myself at home? What are the risks of doing that?

After I remove the skin tags, what should I look for in terms of complications?

Do the removed skin tags need to be sent to a pathologist for further evaluation?

How many skin tags can be removed at once?

Sleep Apnea

Sleep apnea is a medical condition in which air movement through the throat into the lungs is reduced during sleep. This condition may affect a person's daily activities due to impaired sleep but also has been recognized to have an impact on your general health including an increase in blood pressure. Treatment usually involves a machine called CPAP with a face mask (continuous positive airway pressure) that keeps the lungs fully inflated at night.

Top 5 questions-

Are any of my current medications contributing to my sleep apnea?

Do I need additional tests to confirm my diagnosis of sleep apnea?

I have been told that I snore loudly. Should I be tested for sleep apnea?

What is the most likely cause of my sleep apnea?

What restrictions should I follow because I have sleep apnea?

Additional questions you may consider asking-

Are any of the sleep apnea devices portable?

Do you recommend over the counter products for loud snoring?

What are my CPAP settings?

What things should I keep in mind when choosing different sleep apnea devices such as CPAP?

Will changing the position in which I sleep help improve my sleep apnea?

Will weight loss improve my sleep apnea?

Smoking

Smoking is one of the biggest public health problems in the world. Tobacco use includes chewing tobacco and both smoking and chewing tobacco carry the same risk for cancer. Smoking can lead to many health problems like chronic bronchitis, emphysema and lung cancer. Chewing tobacco can cause throat and mouth cancer. Smoking is a difficult habit to break but it can be done with the help of your doctor.

Top 5 questions-

How can I quit smoking?

How long will it take for me to quit?

If I start a medication to quit smoking, will I need it my whole life?

Once I stop smoking, how long will it take for my risk for cancer to drop?

What should I expect when I quit my tobacco use?

Additional questions you may consider asking-

Do you recommend cutting down or just quitting all at once?

Is chewing tobacco as bad as smoking tobacco?

Is smoking cigars or pipes as bad as smoking cigarettes?

What are the risks of inhaling smoke from someone else (second hand smoke)?

What are the risks to my health from smoking or chewing tobacco?

What medications are available to help me quit? Are any of these medications available for free or over the counter?

Stroke

Stroke is a serious medical condition caused by the interruption of blood supply to the brain. Symptoms of stroke may include difficulty walking, speech impairment, vision problems or headaches. Stroke needs urgent medical attention and an untreated stroke can result in permanent impairment and even death.

Top 5 questions-

How can I prevent a future stroke?

How long will it take for my stroke to resolve?

What are my risk factors for getting a stroke?

What treatment do you recommend for my stroke?

Which tests do you recommend to evaluate my stroke?

Additional questions you may consider asking-

Am I candidate for medications that burst the clot causing my stroke?

I had a temporary loss of vision that went away on its own. Can that be a stroke?

What are the possible long-term problems I can have from my stroke?

What can be done to improve the weakness I developed after my stroke?

What is a mini-stroke?

What is my goal blood pressure and cholesterol, now that I had a stroke?

Will I be able to return to work in the same capacity as before my stroke?

Syncope

This condition is commonly known as fainting or passing out. Syncope can be caused by stress, severe pain, low blood pressure, heart problems (such as arrhythmias), dehydration, or seizures. There is a form of syncope called vasovagal syncope that some people call the "fight or flight reflex." In this form of syncope a person can faint as a result of fear. Most syncope is not dangerous, but it will need to be investigated by your doctor to make sure you don't have any medical conditions that could be causing it.

Top 5 questions-

Am I likely to get future episodes of syncope? If yes, how can I prevent them?

Do I need go to the emergency room or get hospitalized for syncope?

What activities should I avoid? Can I drive?

What is the cause of my syncope?

What tests do you recommend to find the cause of my syncope?

Additional questions you may consider asking-

Are any of the medications I take causing syncope?

Do I need to see a specialist (neurologist, cardiologist) for syncope?

I feel faint every time I stand up from a sitting position. What can I do to prevent that?

What is a tilt table test?

What is near syncope?

Temporo-Mandibular Joint Dysfunction (TMJ)

Temporo-mandibular joint dysfunction (TMJ for short) is a common cause of jaw pain. The temporo-mandibular joint is in front of the ears where the lower jaw is attached to the upper part of the face. If you put your hands in front of your ears and open your mouth you can feel the TMJ area move. This joint can develop pain along with difficulty in chewing and biting. TMJ dysfunction may also present with a clicking sound with jaw movements.

Top 5 questions-

Are there medications I can take for the pain?

Do I need a bite guard, and how do I use us it?

Do I need to have any tests like an x-ray or a CAT scan?

I grind my teeth during sleep. Will that lead to TMJ dysfunction?

What causes TMJ dysfunction?

Additional questions you may consider asking-

Are there any jaw exercises you recommend for TMJ dysfunction?

Are there types of food that will cause less jaw pain?

Can my TMJ be treated with botulinum (Botox) injections? How does Botox treat TMJ?

I was prescribed a medication for TMJ which is used to treat depression. Does that mean I am depressed?

Will applying heat to the TMJ area help with the pain?

Tendonitis

Tendons are thick structures that attach muscles to bones. Inflammation of tendons is called tendonitis. Tendonitis is most commonly seen around the shoulders (swimmer's shoulder or rotator cuff tendonitis), elbows (tennis elbow, golfer's elbow) and heels (achilles tendonitis). It presents with pain and swelling at the site of the tendon and is generally caused by repetitive movements of the tendons over time.

Top 5 questions-

How can you tell that I have tendonitis?

Is this tendonitis caused by activities at my job?

What can I do to prevent tendonitis?

What is the cause of my tendonitis? What daily activities could be causing it?

What treatment do you recommend for tendonitis? Will physical therapy and exercises help?

Additional questions you may consider asking-

Do I need to see a specialist (orthopedics or pain specialist)?

Should I apply ice or heat to the area of tendonitis?

What are the risks of having tendinitis?

What is the difference between tendonitis and arthritis?

Which activities should I avoid since I now have tendonitis?

Which pain medications do you recommend my tendonitis?

Thyroid Disorders

The thyroid gland is a butterfly shaped gland located in the lower part of neck and it produces hormones called thyroid hormones (T4 and T3 for short). These hormones are responsible for a variety of body functions including protein production, normal heart function and maintaining a normal energy level in the body. Thyroid disorders include conditions such as hypothyroidism (low levels of thyroid hormone), hyperthyroidism (high levels of thyroid hormone), thyroid nodules and cancer of the thyroid gland. Thyroid surgery and certain medications can also lead to hypothyroidism. Thyroid nodules can lead to hyperthyroidism.

Top 5 questions-

Do I have a hyperactive or hypoactive thyroid?

Do you recommend testing for thyroid disorders even if I don't have any symptoms?

How can my thyroid condition be treated? Do I need to have treatment my whole life?

What are the common symptoms of thyroid disorders?

What is the cause of my thyroid disorder?

Additional questions you may consider asking-

Are there any medications that can affect the absorption of the thyroid supplements I take?

Can thyroid cancer cause hyperactive or hypoactive thyroid?

Do I need to see a specialist (endocrinologist)?

How can we monitor the treatment of my thyroid condition?

I am told that I have high thyroid hormones detected on routine screening but I do not have any symptoms. Do I still need treatment for this?

I am told that I have low thyroid detected on routine screening but I do not have any symptoms. Do I still need treatment for this?

I have depression. Should I get my thyroid hormones checked?

I have heard that iodine is involved in the production of thyroid hormones. Am I getting adequate iodine in my diet?

I have high cholesterol. Should I get my thyroid hormones checked?

What additional tests do I need to further evaluate my thyroid?

What are the possible risks of having hyperactive and hypoactive thyroid?

What is a goiter?

Will a hypoactive thyroid cause weight gain?

Tinea Infection (Fungus Infection)

Tinea is a fungus infection that may involve the skin, hair or nails. There are two common types of tinea. The most common tinea infection is called ringworm (because of the ring-like appearance of the rash) and it may involve any part of your body such as the feet, groin, head, arms, legs or face. Ringworm infection on the feet is called athlete's feet. Infections in the groin area are called jock itch. The other type of tinea infection is called tinea versicolor (pityriasis versicolor) where there are patchy changes in the color of the skin. Tinea infections spread very easily from one person to another (it is contagious).

Top 5 questions-

Can over the counter creams and ointments treat my tinea infection?

How did I get this infection and how can I avoid getting it again?

How do I know I have a tinea infection and not something else?

I have yellow nails due to a tinea infection. How is this treated?

What is the difference between ringworm and a tinea versicolor infection?

Additional questions you may consider asking-

Can sharing gym equipment cause a tinea infection, and how do I avoid it?

How long will it take for the infection to go away after starting treatment?

How often should I apply the cream (or ointment)?

Should I leave the areas of tinea infection dry or moisturized them?

What do I do if the infection is not gone after finishing the cream?

Tinnitus (Ringing in the Ears)

Tinnitus is noise or ringing in the ears. Tinnitus may be caused by conditions such as hearing loss, injury to the ear from loud noise, ear wax, or medications. It may also be caused by medical conditions such as tumors or extra fluid inside the ear.

Top 5 questions-

Are there any over the counter medications I can take for my tinnitus?

How long do you think my tinnitus will last?

What is the cause of my tinnitus?

What tests do you recommend to find the reason for my tinnitus?

Which lifestyle changes do you suggest to treat tinnitus?

Additional questions you may consider asking-

Are any of the medications I take causing my tinnitus?

Do I need to see a specialist (ear, nose and throat doctor)?

How long after removal of my ear wax will tinnitus disappear?

I get exposed to loud noise at work. How can I prevent developing tinnitus?

Tonsillitis

The tonsils are lymph nodes (glands) located deep inside the mouth at the top of the throat. They normally help filter out bacteria and other infectious agents. Tonsillitis is inflammation of the tonsils. It can be caused by a variety of infectious agents such as viruses and bacteria.

Top 5 questions-

Do I need a throat culture (throat swab) to confirm the diagnosis?

Do I need antibiotics to treat my tonsillitis?

Is this episode of tonsillitis contagious (can be spread to other people)?
- If yes, then how long will I be contagious?

What are the possible risks of having tonsillitis?

What is the most likely cause of my tonsillitis?

Additional questions you may consider asking-

Am I allowed to air travel while having tonsillitis?

Am I likely to get this again? If yes, how do I prevent it?

Can this infection involve other body parts (sinuses, heart, kidneys, or liver)?

Can you suggest over the counter medications I can take?

If my tonsillitis happens over and over again, do I need to have them removed?

What medicines can I take to relieve my throat pain?

Tooth Pain

Tooth pain (toothache) is often caused by a dental problem such as a cavity, abscess (infection), cracked tooth or gum problems like gingivitis (inflammation of the gums around the teeth). In some cases a toothache may be caused by problems elsewhere such as in ears, sinuses or heart. This is called referred pain.

Top 5 questions-

Do I need to see a dentist right away?

If untreated, what could be the risk of continuing with my toothache?

What can I do to prevent future toothaches?

What is the cause of my toothache?

What types of pain medications do you recommend for my toothache?

Additional questions you may consider asking-

Hot and cold foods bother my teeth. What does that mean?

How frequently should I visit a dentist for a regular check up?

Which is better to take for tooth pain, ibuprofen (Advil, Motrin) or acetaminophen (Tylenol)?

Tremors

Tremors are uncontrolled small shaking movements of a body part. Most tremors are in the hands, but they may also involve the arms, legs, head, face or trunk. Tremors can be seen in conditions such as anxiety, Parkinson's disease, alcohol use, excess caffeine use, and hyperthyroidism. Certain medications can also cause tremors. The most common type of tremor is called an essential tremor and has no known cause.

Top 5 questions-

If I drink less caffeine will my tremor go away?

My family member has been diagnosed with an essential tremor. How can they prevent it?

What are the treatment choices for my tremor?

What conditions and medications can cause my hands to shake?

Why do I have a tremor?

Additional questions you may consider asking-

Are there alternative treatments like acupuncture for tremors?

Can stopping medication (withdrawal) lead to a tremor?

What is a non-intentional tremor?

Which conditions can make an essential tremor worse?

Will the tremor go away, or will I have it forever? Will it get worse?

Upper Respiratory Infection (URI)

URI is an illness that involves the nose, sinuses, throat and ears. Runny nose, nasal congestion, sore throat, cough, fever and fatigue are some of the features of this condition. URI is also commonly referred to as the common cold and is caused by viruses. Influenza (flu) presents with symptoms similar to a URI, but the flu is likely to have other symptoms such as body aches, nausea, vomiting, diarrhea, and a high fever. Most URIs will resolve in a few days with or without treatment.

Top 5 questions-

Can I go to work while having my URI?

How can I prevent getting another URI?

How long will my URI last?

I get frequent URIs. Why does that happen?

What do you think is causing my URI? Do I have the flu?

Additional questions you may consider asking-

Are antibacterial hand soaps effective in preventing the spread of an URI?

Can I air travel with an URI? If yes, what precautions should I take?

Do I need to see a doctor every time I have an URI?

Do I need to take an antibiotic to treat this URI?

How does an URI spread from person to person?

Which over the counter medications do you suggest for an URI?

Urinary Tract Infection (UTI)

Urinary tract infections (UTI for short) are more common in women than men. UTIs happen when germs (bacteria) get into the urethra (the tube that you urinate through). The most common bacteria that cause a UTI is E. Coli (the bacteria in stool). UTIs cause dysuria (burning when urinating) and usually require treatment with antibiotics in order to go away.

Top 5 questions-

Do I need any special tests to see if the infection is in my kidneys?

How can I prevent getting another UTI?

What, in your opinion, caused my UTI?

What are the most common reasons for getting a UTI?

What is the result of my urine culture and urinalysis (urine test)? What bacteria were found?

Additional questions you may consider asking-

Are any medications I am taking affecting my urinary system?

Did I get a urinary tract infection from my sexual partner?

How much water should I normally drink?

How will I know if my treatment is working?

Is my UTI contagious?

Will drinking cranberry juice help?

Vasculitis

Vasculitis is inflammation of the blood vessels. It can be caused by infections, diseases of the connective tissue (such as lupus, scleroderma, and rheumatoid arthritis), allergic reactions and cancer. The symptoms of vasculitis can be tiredness, lack of appetite, joint pain or weight loss. Some forms of vasculitis are hereditary (run in the family).

Top 5 questions-

Can my vasculitis go away with treatment?

Does vasculitis run in the family?

How do you determine that I have vasculitis?

What is the cause of my vasculitis?

What treatments do you recommend for my vasculitis?

Additional questions you may consider asking-

Do I need to see a specialist (vascular surgeon)?

If a medicine caused my vasculitis and I stop it, how long will it take to get better?

What are the possible risks of having vasculitis?

What can I do prevent vasculitis?

Which blood vessels are involved in my vasculitis?

Which body parts are involved in my vasculitis?

Venous Insufficiency

Chronic venous insufficiency is a medical condition where blood pools in the veins of the lower legs. People who are obese, extremely inactive, or elderly may develop this condition because all three factors can lead to problems with the valves in the veins. Venous insufficiency can also be inherited. The symptoms of venous insufficiency are ankle and leg swelling. The diagnosis is made by a history and physical and sometimes a procedure called a duplex scanning (doppler), which is a painless ultrasound of the veins. Treatment for venous insufficiency includes compression stockings worn on the legs which squeeze the veins to keep blood flowing. Elevation of the legs and medications are also a common treatment.

Top 5 questions-

Am I at risk for an infection (leg ulcer or cellulitis)?

Do I need a duplex scanning examination (doppler)?

How can I prevent an infection?

How often should I wear the compression stockings and for how long?

Why is it important to elevate my legs above my heart?

Additional questions you may consider asking-

Can I take over the counter or prescription medication for the pain?

Do I need to see a specialist (vascular surgeon)?

Will a daily aspirin help my circulation?

Will regular exercise and weight loss help my circulation?

Venous Thromboembolism (Blood Clots)

Venous thromboembolism is a medical term for clots that form in blood vessels called veins. These clots usually happen in the deeper blood vessels of the legs (deep venous thrombosis), but they can happen in any vein. Sometimes these clots can travel to the lungs and cause a pulmonary embolism (clot in the lung) which is a very serious condition. People with clots in their legs will have leg swelling and pain and people with clots in their lungs may feel short of breath or experience chest pain. Obesity (being overweight), older age, tobacco use, traveling long distances, surgery, immobilization, birth control pills and certain familial conditions can increase your risk for venous thromboembolism.

Top 5 questions-

Do I need to be hospitalized to manage this clot or can I be treated in the doctor's office?

How can I prevent a future clot?

Can this clot be removed by surgery?

How long do I need to be on a blood thinner (medication that prevents clots) to treat this clot?

What is my risk of getting another clot if I stop taking the blood thinner?

Additional questions you may consider asking-

Am I at risk for getting more clots?

Can I ever stop taking the blood thinner?

Do any of the medications I take cause clots?

Do I need to see a specialist (vascular surgeon)?

Do my family members need to be tested for a blood clot?

Is the venous clot I have restricted to my legs and arms or has it spread to my lungs?

Is there a routine test that can be performed to check for clots? How is that test performed?

What are my risk factors for getting a venous clot?

What are some of the risks of having venous clots?

What dietary restrictions should I follow if I am on a blood thinner medication?

What tests should I have to determine my risk for future clots?

What things do you suggest I do to avoid future venous clots?

Would I benefit from a filter that blocks travel of the clot from my legs to my lungs (Greenfield filter)?

Will exercise help decrease my risks of getting venous clots?

Will weight loss decrease my risk of getting venous clots?

Vitamin B 12 Deficiency

Vitamin B 12 (cobalamin) is an essential vitamin found in a variety of foods such as fish, meat and dairy products. It is involved in maintaining healthy nerve function and production of red blood cells. Low levels of vitamin B 12 can result from inadequate intake of those foods, or medical conditions such as malabsorption and pernicious anemia. In many cases, this condition may remain without any symptoms and only be detected as part of a routine blood test.

Top 5 questions-

Am I at risk to develop vitamin B 12 deficiency?

Can I take over the counter vitamin B 12 supplements?

What are some of the risks of having a vitamin B 12 deficiency?

What is the cause of my vitamin B 12 deficiency?

Which foods are rich in vitamin B 12?

Additional questions you may consider asking-

Can a vitamin B 12 deficiency lead to dementia?

Do I need any medical tests now that I have been diagnosed with a vitamin B 12 deficiency?

Does drinking alcohol lead to low vitamin B 12 levels?

How is the diagnosis of vitamin B 12 deficiency made?

What are normal levels for vitamin B 12?

What is pernicious anemia?

Vitamin D Deficiency

Vitamin D is required for a variety of body functions including maintaining healthy bones. A lot of attention has been given to vitamin D recently, as its role in reducing inflammation and improving cardiovascular health are being increasingly recognized. Your body makes its own supply of vitamin D (in the skin) from exposure to sunlight. This vitamin is also present in foods such as fish and milk. People with deficiency of this vitamin may be completely without any symptoms or they may have complications such as thin bones, high blood pressure, and chronic pain, or symptoms of muscle aches or fatigue.

Top 5 questions-

How can my vitamin D deficiency be corrected?

Should I be taking an over the counter vitamin D supplement?

What are some of the best food sources of Vitamin D?

What is a normal level of vitamin D, and what is my level?

Why do you think I have a vitamin D deficiency?

Additional questions you may consider asking-

Do you recommend routine testing for vitamin D deficiency?

I am a vegan. Does that put me at a high risk for vitamin D deficiency?

If I have osteoporosis, should I be taking vitamin D supplements?

I take a multivitamin daily. Does that have adequate amounts of vitamin D to prevent deficiency?

Why doesn't my body absorb vitamin D like it should?

Warts (Common Wart)

Warts are a common skin condition. They are initially started by a virus on the skin, but the wart itself (the raised area of skin) can remain long after the body has fought off the virus. If a wart doesn't go away after a long period of time, or hurts, or if multiple warts occur, your doctor may apply a freezing medication to the wart to kill the raised area of skin or may suggest cryotherary (burning the wart).

Top 5 questions-

Am I contagious (can pass this to someone else)?

If I leave the wart alone will it go away?

Is my wart a sign of any other medical condition?

What are my treatment options?

Will Compound W (an over the counter treatment) work on my wart?

Additional questions you may consider asking-

Do I need to see a specialist (dermatologist)?

If I get a wart in my genital area (private area), does that mean I have a sexually transmitted disease?

Is it dangerous to cut the wart off myself with a razor?

What should I expect after you treat my wart?

Index

E

F

D

K

kidney failure · 50
kidney stone · 71, 101
kidneys · 11, 32, 37, 50, 65, 143, 147

L

labyrinthitis · 72
lactose intolerance · 67
latex · 64
laxative · 57
LDL cholesterol · 91
Legionnaires' disease · 124
leukemia · 102
Lewy body dementia · 61
LFT's · 104
lipoma · 103
lithotripsy · 101
liver failure · 52
liver function tests · 14, 104
low platelet count · 38
lupus · 24, 26, 64, 106, 148
lupus arthritis · 26
Lyme disease · 105

M

malignant · 43
memory loss · 61
meningitis · 107
menopause · 108
menorrhagia · 74
menstrual cycle · 70
menstruation · 18, 70, 74
metabolic syndrome · 109
metastasis · 43
migraine · 39, 110
mitral valve prolapse · 111
Motrin · 144
murmur · 111
myocardial infarction · 112
myopia · 39

N

nausea · 11, 22, 70, 80, 82, 102, 110, 114, 119, 146
neck pain · 20, 115
nicotine · 99, 118
nitroglycerin · 19, 112, 113
nits · 86
non-HDL cholesterol · 91
Non-Tropical Sprue · 45
nummular dermatitis · 64
nutrition · 77

O

obesity · 46, 64, 87, 116
osteoarthritis · 24
osteoporosis · 93, 108, 117, 153
otitis externa · 72
otitis media · 72

P

pacemaker · 23
palpitations · 23, 111, 118
palsy · 36
pancreas · 32, 65, 119
pancreatitis · 119
paralysis · 36
Parkinson's dementia · 61
Parkinson's disease · 64, 120, 121, 145
patch test · 64, 85
PCOS · 90
pediculosis · 86
pelvic inflammatory disease · 70
peripheral vascular disease · 29
pharyngitis · 122
photophobia · 110
physical therapy · 20, 24, 32, 115, 138
pink eye · 56
pituitary gland · 16
pityriasis versicolor · 141
plantar fasciitis · 123
plaques · 10
pneumonia · 28, 40, 58, 124
pneumonia shot · 28
poison ivy · 64
Polycystic ovarian syndrome · 90

URI · 146
uric acid · 84
urinalysis · 71
urinary tract infection · 71, 101, 147
urine · 37, 50, 71, 101, 147
UTI · 147

V

vascular dementia · 61
vasculitis · 38, 148
vasovagal syncope · 136
venous insufficiency · 149
venous thromboembolism · 150
vertigo · 69
virtual colonoscopy · 53
vitamin B 12 deficiency · 152
vitamin D · 20, 93, 117, 153
vitamin D deficiency · 93, 153

vitamins · 45
vomiting · 22, 80, 82, 102, 114, 119, 146
Von Willebrand disease · 38

W

warfarin · 23, 38
warts · 154
wheezing · 28

X

x-ray · 24, 40, 41, 57, 58, 71, 124, 128, 137

CPSIA information can be obtained at www.ICGtesting.com
Printed in the USA
BVOW061225090312

284833BV00001B/56/P